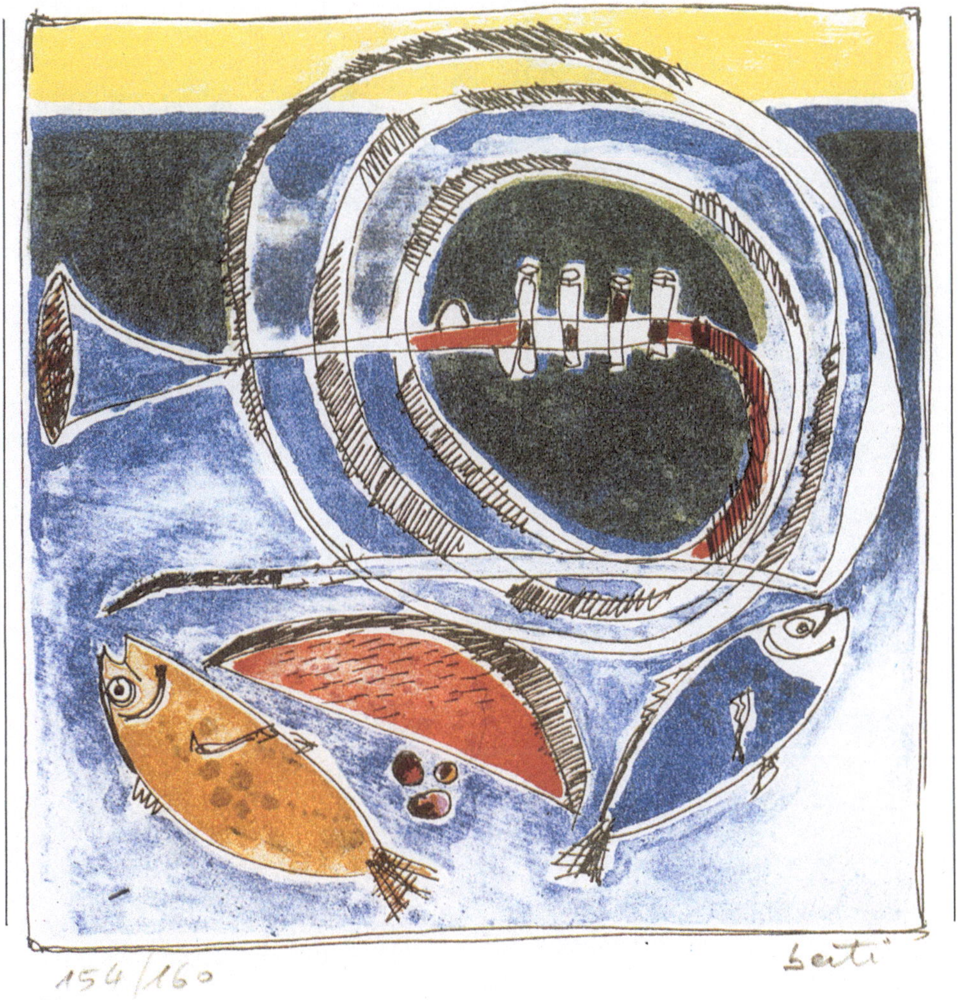

154/160

berti

By courtesy of Alberto Berti, Pisa, Italy

Fish Oil and
Vascular Disease

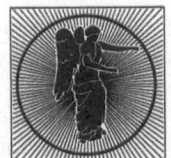

Bi & Gi Publishers

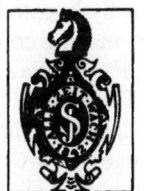

Current Topics in Cardiovascular Diseases
Series Editor: G. Crepaldi M.D.

Title in the series:

Fish Oil and Vascular Disease
Edited by: R. De Caterina, S.D. Kristensen, E.B. Schmidt

Acknowledgments: This book contains the proceedings of the oral presentations from the first workshop on *Fish oil and Vascular disease* that was held in Pisa, Italy, 3-6 April 1991, within the framework of the European Society of Clinical Investigation and was published with a grant from Farmitalia Carlo Erba.
The general annual meeting of the European Society of Investigation attracts scientists and clinicians working in other areas and the large, unexpected attendance to the workshop has certainly boosted our enthusiasm in editing this book.
This meeting could not have been arranged without the support of the following contributors: Farmitalia-Carlo Erba, Italy (main sponsor), Ciba-Geigy, Italy, Norsk Hydro, Norway and Peter Møller, Norway.
We hope that the book will stimulate more research in the n-3 area and look forward to arrange a new workshop on *Fish oil and vascular disease* at the 27th annual meeting of the European Society of Clinical Investigation in Heidelberg in 1993.

Fish Oil and Vascular Disease

Edited by: R. De Caterina, S.D. Kristensen, E.B. Schmidt

Foreword by: G. Crepaldi
With 43 figures and 32 tables

Springer-Verlag London Ltd.

R. De Caterina	- C.N.R. Institute of Clinical Physiology, Pisa, Italy
S.D. Kristensen	- University Department of Cardiology, Skejby Hospital, Aarhus, Denmark
E.B. Schmidt	- Department of Internal Medicine, Aalborg Hospital, Aalborg, Denmark

Series Editor:
G. Crepaldi   - Institute of Internal Medicine, University of Padua, Italy

ISBN 978-1-4471-3892-1

British Library Cataloguing in Publication Data
Fish Oil and Vascular Disease - (Current Topics in Cardiovascular Diseases Series) I. Caterina, R. De. II. Series 616.1
ISBN 978-1-4471-3892-1   ISBN 978-1-4471-3890-7 (eBook)
DOI 10.1007/978-1-4471-3890-7

Library of Congress Cataloging in Publication Data
Fish oil and vascular disease/edited by R. De Caterina. S.D. Kristensen E.B. Schmidt: foreword by G. Crepaldi p. cm. -- (Topics in cardiovascular diseases)
Includes bibliographical references and index ISBN 978-1-4471-3892-1
1. Atherosclerosis -- Prevention. 2. Omega-3 fatty acids -- Health aspects. 3. Fish oils in human nutrition. 4. Cardiovascular system -- Diseases -- Nutritional aspects. I. De Caterina. R., 1954 - II. Kristensen, S.D. 1955- Schmidt, E.B., 1952- IV Series. (DNLM 1 Fish Oils--metabolism. 2. Fish Oils--therapeutic use. 3. Vascular Diseases--diet therapy. 4. Vascular Diseases--prevention & control. WG 500 F532) RC692. F48 1992
616.1 '360654--dc20 DNLM/DLC 92-49797 CIP for Library of Congress
©1992 Springer-Verlag London
Originally published by Springer-Verlag London Berlin Heidelberg New York in 1992
Softcover reprint of the hardcover 1st edition 1992

Typeset by Bi & Gi, Verona, Italy

Foreword

Cardiovascular diseases are the leading cause of morbility and mortality in the affluent societies of the western world. This simple statement should justify every possible effort to treat or (even better) to prevent such a social disease. On the contrary, we are often impressed by the great deal of scientific and economic energies devoted to some specific (but often limited in terms of epidemiological involvement) health problems.

I would greatly recommend to start from the basic point: the patients. Our clinics, our hospitals are all too often crowded by patients with vascular diseases in many of whom the vascular event was fully preventable. We believe that it remains for physicians to take care of the preventive strategies for vascular disease.

With these thoughts in our mind as physicians we spent most of our time looking for an effective prevention of vascular diseases by studying patients with risk factors for these diseases. With this background we reached the conclusion that both primary and secondary prevention of vascular diseases are worth to pursuing. Of course, we are willing to discuss which is the best approach to this prevention in a never ending search for better options.

Along this line *Current topics in cardiovascular disease is* aimed to address as many topics as possible to update and highlight the scientific basis of the biological, pathological, diagnostic, and therapeutic approaches to cardiovascular disease.

These volumes, as they will grow in the near future, should allow researchers and clinicians to find easily a large body of references about specific topics. We hope that this editorial endeavour will be rewarded by the interest and possibly the contributions of as many readers and workers as possible in this field.

June 1992

GAETANO CREPALDI

Preface

In 1978 Dyerberg and Bang suggested that the high content of n-3 polyunsaturated fatty acids present in the traditional Eskimo food was offering protection against atherosclerosis and thrombosis. This has inspired several other groups to do epidemiological investigations on the importance of dietary intake of fish and to explore the effects of n-3 polyunsaturated fatty acids on various important biological systems. Within the last five years the effects of dietary supplementation with n-3 polyunsaturated fatty acids have been evaluated in clinical studies in various groups of patients. The purpose of this book is to present recent important results in these areas and to provide stimulating discussions between clinicians and basic scientists.

This book is divided into three main sections. The first deals with the epidemiological and nutritional background of the n-3 polyunsaturated fatty acids (PUFA) and their relation to cardiovascular disease. The second section is devoted to n-3 PUFA and the vessel wall, with particular focus on the possible mechanisms by which n-3 PUFA may work as anti-atherosclerotic agents. The third and final section deals with n-3 PUFA and blood pressure - an area of controversy that may have settled down after the completion of two recent prospective trials.

It is evident that n-3 PUFA have several levels of interaction in various biological systems that may be important in atherogenesis and thrombogenesis. This multiplex action is probably what makes n-3 PUFA so interesting at a time when cardiovascular science is exploring major areas such as prevention and treatment of atherogenesis and its complications, thrombosis and tissue damage. The traditional strategy is to develop specific pharmacological agents to attack a single pathway.

It seems that n-3 PUFA, in a more comprehensive strategy, have pharmacological effects in several important biological systems.

We hope that this book will stimulate more research in the various areas of biology and clinical applications of n-3 fatty acids which still need to be investigated.

R. De Caterina
S.D. Kristensen
E.B. Schmidt

Contents

X

Contributors

K.H. Bønaa
Institute of Community Medicine, University of Tromsø, Breivika, Norway

M.L. Burr
MRC Epidemiological Unit, Llandough Hospital, Penarth, South Glamorgan, UK

S. Colli
Institute of Pharmacological Sciences, E. Grossi Paoletti Center, University of Milan, Milan, Italy

R. De Caterina
CNR Institute of Clinical Physiology, Pisa, Italy

J. Dyerberg
Medi-Lab a.s., Copenhagen, Denmark

S. Eligini
Institute of Pharmacological Sciences, E. Grossi Paoletti Center, University of Milan, Milan, Italy

S. Endres
Medizinische Klinik, Klinikum Innenstadt der Universitat, Munich, Federal Republic of Germany

G.A. FitzGerald
Center for Cardiovascular Sciences, Department of Medicine and Experimental Therapeutics, University College Dublin, Mater Hospital, Dublin, Ireland

C. Galli
Institute of Pharmacological Sciences, E. Grossi Paoletti Center, University of Milan, Milan, Italy

H. Hallaq
Medical Services, Massachusetts General Hospital, Boston, Massachusetts, USA

G. Hornstra
Department of Human Biology, Limburg University, Maastricht, The Netherlands

XII

P.R. Jackson
University Department of Medicine and Therapeutics, Royal Hallamshire Hospital, Sheffield, UK

S.D. Kristensen
University Department of Cardiology, Skejby Hospital, Aarhus, Denmark

A. Leaf
Medical Services, Massachusetts General Hospital, Boston, Massachusetts, USA

P. Maderna
Institute of Pharmacological Sciences, E. Grossi Paoletti Center, University of Milan, Milan, Italy

C. Mosconi
Institute of Pharmacological Sciences, E. Grossi Paoletti Center, University of Milan, Milan, Italy

A. Nordøy
Department of Medicine, Tromsø University Hospital, Tromsø, Norway

L.E. Ramsay
University Department of Medicine and Therapeutics, Royal Hallamshire Hospital, Sheffield, UK

E.B. Schmidt
Department of Medicine II, Aalborg Hospital, Danimarca; Department of Medicine, Section of Clinical Nutrition, Oregon Health Sciences University, Portland, Oregon, USA

A.P. Simopoulos
The Center for Genetics, Nutrition and Health, Washington DC, USA

P. Singer
Stoffwechselklinik Lindenfels,Federal Republic of Germany

C. Sirtori
Institute of Pharmacological Sciences, E. Grossi Paoletti Center, University of Milan, Milan, Italy

E. Stragliotto
Institute of Pharmacological Sciences, E. Grossi Paoletti Center, University of Milan, Milan, Italy

E. Tremoli
Institute of Pharmacological Sciences, E. Grossi Paoletti Center, University of Milan, Milan, Italy

B.B. WEKSLER
Division of Hematology-Oncology, Department of Medicine, Cornell University Medical College, New York, USA

W.W. YEO
University Department of Medicine and Therapeutics, Royal Hallamshire Hospital, Sheffield, UK

XIII

S.D. Horton
Division of Hematology/Oncology, Department of Medicine, Cornell University Medical College, New York, USA

W.W. Yeo
Department of Medicine and Therapeutics, Royal Hallamshire Hospital, Sheffield, UK

Epidemiology and Nutrition

1. n-3 Fatty Acids: Epidemiological Background and General Introduction

J. DYERBERG

Medi-Lab a.s. Copenhagen, Denmark

Coronary Heart Disease in Greenland Eskimos

The mortality from coronary heart disease is low in Greenland Eskimos compared to Western populations.[1,2] The fact that this difference also exists, though not to the extent found in Eskimos, in comparison with other populations with a habitually high intake of sea-food suggests that dietary habits are responsible for this finding.[3,4]

A careful analysis of the Eskimo diet[5] has shown that the main difference compared to the Western diet lies in an extremely high intake of n-3 fatty acids derived from sea food in the Eskimos (Tab. I). A causal relationship between a high dietary intake of n-3 fatty acids and a low mortality from coronary heart disease has therefore been hypothesized.[6]

Fatty Acids: Types and Characteristics

To better understand the basis of this relationship it is necessary to review some basic notions concerning n-3 fatty acids. First, there are several classes of fatty acids: saturated, monounsaturated and polyunsaturated, based on the number of double bonds in the aliphatic chain. In figure 1 examples of these three types of fatty acids are shown.

Each class of fatty acid has different properties and unique biological effects and roles.[7] Among the polyunsaturated fatty acids two distinct classes (n-3 and n-6) have been shown to play a major role in modulating cell function and cell reactivity

Table I. Dietary fats in the food of Greenland Eskimos and in Danish controls. Values are computed on a daily energy consumption of 3000 kcal.

		Eskimos	Danes
Fat Energy %		**39**	**42**
Saturated:	12:2	1.1	5.9
	14:0	3.7	7.5
	16:0	13.6	25.5
	18:0	4.0	9.5
	20:0	0.1	4.3
	Total	**23**	**53**
Monoenes:	16:1	9.8	3.8
	18:1	24.6	29.2
	20:1	14.7	0.4
	22:1	8.0	1.2
	Total	**58**	**34**
Polyenes:	18:2n-6	5.0	10.0
	18:3n-3	0.6	2.0
	20:5n-3	4.6	0.5
	22.5n-3	2.6	0
	22:6n-3	5.9	0.3
	Total	**19**	**13**
P/S ratio		**0.84**	**0.24**
n-3 PUFAs (g/day)		**14**	**3**
n-6 PUFAs (g/day)		**5**	**10**
Cholesterol (g/day)		**0.79**	**0.42**

to external stimuli.[8] The position of the double bond defines polyunsaturated fatty acids as n-6 or n-3.

If the first double bond is located at carbon atom number 3 as counted from the methyl end, the fatty acid belongs to the n-3 type.

In contrast, the first double bond is placed at carbon atom number 6 in n-6 polyunsaturated fatty acids. Both linoleic acid and alpha-linolenic acid, the precursors of the n-6 and the n-3 classes, respectively, are essential fatty acids because the human organism is not able to synthesize them from other classes of fatty acids.

The n-6 and n-3 classes of fatty acids are both fundamental components of cytoplasmic membranes. Also, their metabolism leads to generation of eicosanoids, that are very important intercellular mediators of a series of cellular reactions.

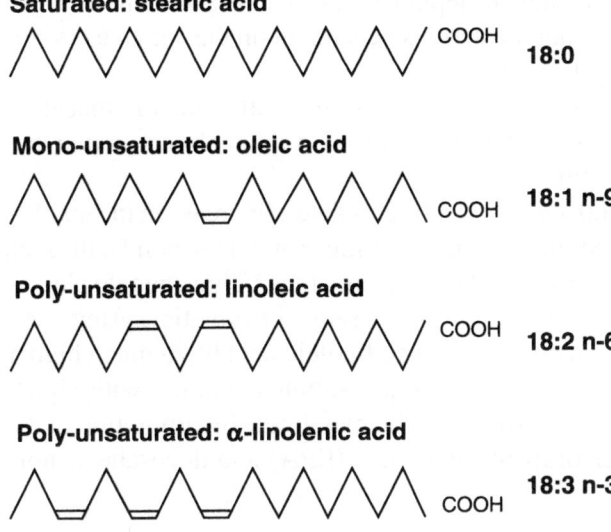

Saturated: stearic acid

COOH 18:0

Mono-unsaturated: oleic acid

COOH 18:1 n-9

Poly-unsaturated: linoleic acid

COOH 18:2 n-6

Poly-unsaturated: α-linolenic acid

COOH 18:3 n-3

Fig. 1. Examples of a saturated fatty acid (stearic acid), a monounsaturated fatty acid (oleic acid) and a polyunsaturated fatty acid of the n-6 class (linoleic acid) and of the n-3 class (alpha-linolenic acid) are shown. To the right, the number of carbon atoms is given before the colon and the number of double bonds after the colon.

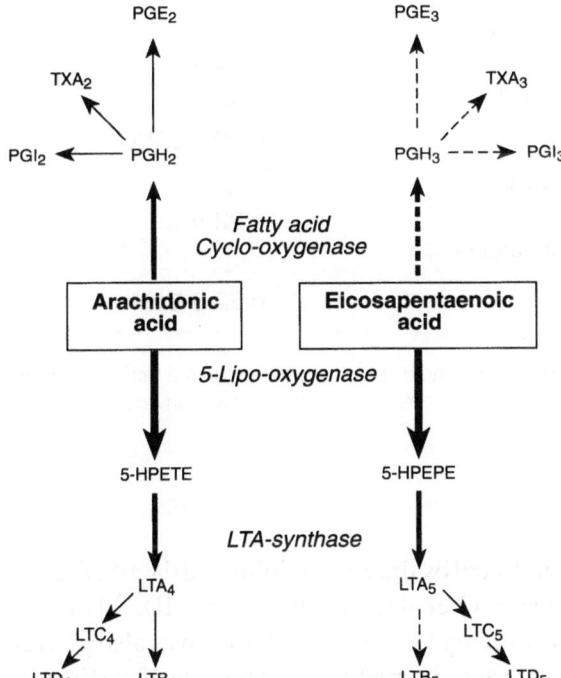

Fig. 2. The metabolism of the n-6 fatty acid arachidonic acid and the n-3 fatty acid eicosapentaenoic acid to eicosanoids is shown.

6

Indeed, prostaglandins, thromboxanes and leukotrienes all derive from the metabolism of n-3 and n-6 fatty acids through reactions dependent on the enzymes cyclo-oxygenase and lipo-oxygenase (Fig. 2).

Another very important characteristic of n-3 and n-6 fatty acids is that their metabolism is completely separated, since a n-3 fatty acid cannot be converted into a n-6 fatty acid and vice versa (Fig. 3).

However, fatty acids from both classes can be elongated (increase in the number of carbon atoms) and desaturated (increase in the number of double bonds) through each pathway by processes catalyzed by the same enzymes.[9] Thus the two classes of polyunsaturated fatty acids compete for the same enzymatic system. An important implication of this concept is that since linoleic acid has a much higher affinity for the delta-6 desaturase enzyme, dietary supplementation with alpha-linolenic acid is not sufficient per se to increase the membrane incorporation of the long chained n-3 derivatives eicosapentaenoic acid (EPA) and docosahexaenoic acid (DHA).[10]

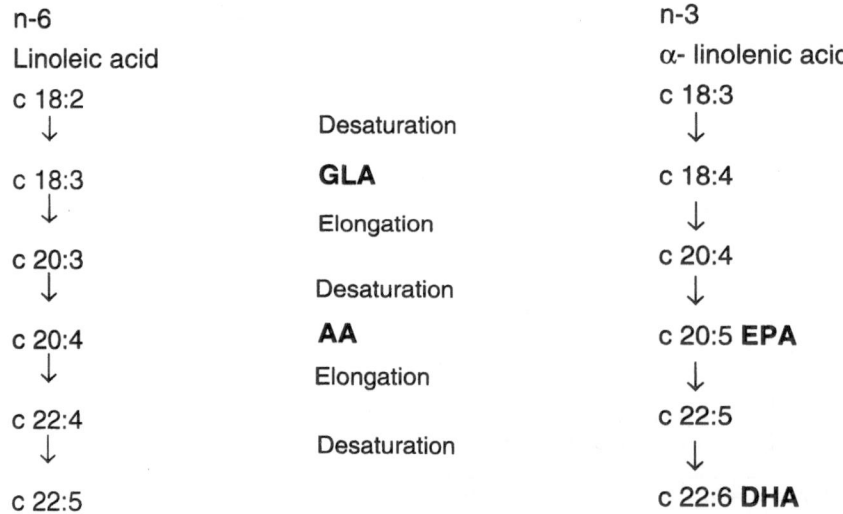

Fig. 3. The elongation and desaturation of the n-6 fatty acid linoleic acid and the n-3 fatty acid alpha-linolenic acid are shown. Note that the same enzymes are used, and that interconversion between classes is not possible.

Epidemiology

The interest in n-3 fatty acids was initiated by the epidemiological data on the low mortality from cardiovascular diseases in Greenland Eskimos (Tab. II).[1,2] This low prevalence of cardiovascular diseases among Greenland Eskimos was also present when subjects were stratified for sex and age.[11] A meticulous analysis of the Eskimo

Table II. Ischaemic heart disease (IHD) rates in Greenland Eskimos compared to those in USA and in Denmark. Results are given for males aged 45-64 years in 1974-78.

IHD deaths/thousand	USA 40.4	Denmark 34.7	Greenland 5.3

Table III. The disease pattern in Greenland Eskimos compared to Western (Scandinavian) citizens.[1]

	Eskimos	:	Scandinavians
Apoplexy	2	:	1
AMI	1	:	10
Psoriasis	1	:	20
Diabetes	Rare		Rare
Bronchial Asthma	1	:	25
Thyreotoxicosis	Rare		Rare
Multiple Sclerosis	0		0
Epilepsy	2	:	1
Polyarthritis Chronica	Low		Low

diet (Tab. I) has highlighted the differences with Western diets, and indeed the high intake of n-3 fatty acids is the most striking difference. Additional data have shown that not only is the incidence of myocardial infarction (1:10) much lower than in typical Western countries, but also that several other diseases are less frequent in Greenland (Tab. III).

The analysis of the epidemiological data available so far indicates that the majority of the studies relating fish consumption to cardiovascular disease without correcting for covariates, that means without adjustment for possible confounding factors, have shown a significant inverse relationship. When data were corrected for these factors in more recent studies, the results have been more controversial.[12,13]

An important contribution in this field has recently been derived from the MRFIT study.[14] In this study, a significant inverse relation between intake of fish and cardiovascular mortality and morbidity has been reported for a very large cohort of subjects also after adjusting for covariates. Very interesting too are the impressive findings from the DART study[15] demonstrating a reduced cardiovascular mortality of 29 % in a secondary prevention study in more than 2000 British men who survived an acute myocardial infarction.

8

Conclusion

These data appear as solid evidence for a protective role of n-3 fatty acids in cardiovascular disease. Several mechanisms may mediate this protective effect. When the beneficial role of n-3 fatty acids was first suggested, the effect on lipids and later on platelet aggregation was believed to be most important. However, more recent data have demonstrated that the mechanisms of action of n-3 fatty acids are multiple and may most likely act synergistically to obtain the beneficial effect.

A definitive demonstration of a preventive effect on cardiovascular disease of a high intake of n-3 fatty acids, however, requires interventional clinical trials targeted to answer this important question.

References

1. Kromann N., Green A.: Epidemiological studies in the Upernavik district, Greenland. Acta Med. Scan. 1980; 208: 401-406
2. Dyerberg J., Bjerregaard P.: Mortality from ischaemic heart disease and cerebrovascular disease in Greenland. In: Lands WEM (Ed) *Proceeding of the AOCS short course in polyunsaturated fatty acids and eicosanoids.* Amer. Oil Chem. Soc. Campaign 111 1987: 2-8
3. Hirai A., Tamura Y.: EPA and adult disease in Japan. n-3 News 1987; 2: 1-3
4. Hirai A., Terano T., Tamura Y., Yoshida S.: Eicosapentaenoic acid and adult disease in Japan: Epidemiological and clinical aspects. J. Intern. Med. 1989; 225 Suppl. 1: 69-75
5. Bang H.O., Dyerberg J., Sinclair H.M.: The composition of the Eskimo food in north western Greenland. Am. J. Clin. Nutr. 1980; 33: 2657-2661
6. Dyerberg J., Bang H.O., Stoffersen E., Moncada S., Vane J.R.: Eicosapentaenoic acid and prevention of thrombosis and atherosclerosis. Lancet 1978; 2: 117-119
7. Nordoy A., Goodnight S.H.: Dietary lipids and thrombosis. Relationships to atherosclerosis. Arteriosclerosis 1990; 10: 149-163
8. Willis A.L.: Nutritional and pharmacological factors in eicosanoid biology. Nutr. Rev. 1981; 39: 289-301
9. Sprecher H.: Interactions between the metabolism of n-3 and n-6 fatty acids. J. Intern. Med. 1989; 225 Suppl. 1: 5-9
10. Dyerberg J., Bang H.O., Aagaard O.: Alfa-Linolenic acid and eicosapentaenoic acid. Lancet 1980; 1: 199
11. Bjerregaard P., Dyerberg J.: Mortality from ischaemic heart disease and cerebrovascular disease in Greeland. Int. J. Epidemiol. 1988; 17: 514-519
12. Kromhout D.: n-3 fatty acids and coronary heart disease: Epidemiology from Eskimos to western populations. J. Intern. Med. 1989; 225 Suppl. 1: 47-51
13. Combie I.K., McLoone P., Smith W.C.S., Thomson M., Pedoe H.T.: International differences in coronary heart disease mortality and consumption of fish and other foodstuffs. European Heart J. 1987; 8: 560-563
14. Dolecek T.A., Grandits G.: Dietary polyunsaturated fatty acids and mortality in the Multiple Risk Factor Intervention Trial (MRFIT). In: Simopoulos A.P., Kifer R.R., Barlow S.M. (Eds.): *Health effects of ω3 polyunsaturated fatty acids in seafoods.* World Rev. Nutr. Diet. Basle, Karger, 1991; 66: 205-215
15. Burr M.L., Fehily A.M., Gilbert J.F., Rogers S., Holliday R.M., Sweetnam P.M., Elwood P.C., Deadman N.M.: Effects of changes in fat, fish and fibre intakes on death and myocardial reinfarction: Diet and reinfarction trial (DART). Lancet 1989; 2: 757-61

2. Dietary Fish Intake and Cardiovascular Protection in Western Populations: the Diet and Reinfarction Trial

M. L. BURR

MRC Epidemiology Unit, Llandough Hospital, Penarth, South Glamorgan, UK

Several studies have suggested that dietary consumption of fish confers some protection against ischaemic heart disease (IHD). The Zutphen study[1] involved a 20-year follow-up of men whose dietary intake had been recorded in detail: those who ate fish regularly had a substantially lower IHD mortality than those who did not (Tab. I). Other cohort studies have shown conflicting results, some showing evidence of a protective effect of fish[2,3] while others have not.[4,5] In general, it seems that a difference in IHD mortality is shown in studies which compare a moderate intake of fish with no fish consumption, but not in studies comparing a high intake with a moderate intake, nor in those where the low-intake group is imprecisely defined (e.g. in terms of a single 24-hour period). Table II shows the findings of the

Table I. Fish consumption and IHD mortality: the Zutphen study

Fish consumption (g/day)	No. subjects	Risk ratio	
		unadjusted	adjusted*
0	159	1.00	1.00
1-14	283	0.60	0.64
15-29	215	0.57	0.56
30-44	116	0.46	0.36
≥45	79	0.42	0.39

p<0 . 0 5; *adjusted for various risk factors

Table II. Fish consumption and coronary mortality: the Western Electric Study

Fish consumption (g/day)	No. subjects	Coronary deaths	
		No.	%
0	205	42	20.5
1-17	686	128	18.7
18-34	779	121	15.5
≥35	261	34	13.0

p<0.01

Western Electric Study,[2] which contained a group eating virtually no fish. Like the Zutphen study, it showed an inverse association between fish intake and mortality.

If fish indeed protects against IHD, it is likely that the effect is attributable to its content of n-3 polyunsaturated fatty acids (PUFA) such as eicosapentaenoic acid (EPA). These fatty acids are known to alter platelet function[6] and serum triglyceride concentrations[7] in ways which are consistent with protection against IHD. The n-3 fatty acids are particularly plentiful in oily fish such as mackerel, herring, salmon, trout, sardine and pilchard.

A randomized controlled trial was set up to see whether an increased intake of fatty fish reduces mortality in men who have recently recovered from myocardial infarction and are therefore at high risk.[8]

A total of 2,033 non-diabetic subjects were admitted to the trial, all under the age of 70 years. The subjects were randomly divided into two groups. Half were advised to eat fatty fish at least twice a week, so as to achieve an intake of 300g weekly; those unable to consume this amount of fish were given fish oil capsules as a partial or total replacement.

The other half of the subjects were given no advice relating to fish. The trial had a factorial design, such that, independently of the randomization for fish advice, half the subjects were advised to reduce their fat intake and increase the proportion of PUFAs, and (independently of fish and fat randomizations) half were advised to increase their intake of cereal fibre. There were thus 8 subgroups of the various combinations of the three types of dietary advice, including a group given no dietary advice at all.

Compliance with fish advice was good, as indicated by dietary questionnaires, and this was confirmed in a subset of subjects by measurement of plasma fatty acids (Tab. III). Subjects who had been given fish advice had higher mean EPA plasma levels than subjects not given that advice.

Table IV shows the deaths occurring within two years of entry into the trial. All-cause mortality was significantly lower in the group given fish advice compared

Table III. Plasma EPA in two dietary advice groups in Diet and Reinfarction Trial

Dietary group	No. subjects	Plasma EPA as % geometric mean	Total fatty acids 95% confidence interval
Fish advice	107	0.59	0.52 - 0.67
No fish advice	96	0.46	0.41 - 0.51

p<0.01

Table IV. Deaths and reinfarctions in relation to fish advice in Diet and Reinfarction Trial

Dietary group	No. subjects	All deaths No. (%)	IHD deaths No. (%)	Non-fatal infarcts No. (%)	IHD events No. (%)
Fish advice	1015	94 (9.3)	78 (7.7)	49 (4.8)	127 (12.5)
No fish advice	1018	130 (12.8)	116 (11.4)	33 (3.2)	149 (14.6)
		p<0.05	p<0.01		

with the rest. This was attributable to a reduction in IHD deaths. There was no reduction in the incidence of non-fatal myocardial infarction.

Table V shows the effects of each of the dietary interventions on the risk of death. The risk ratios are shown before and after adjustment for minor imbalances in the groups regarding certain factors in the histories, x-ray appearances and treatment

Table V. Effects of dietary interventions on death (Diet and Reinfarction Trial)

Dietary intervention	Risk ratio			Significance level
	unadjusted	(95% confidence interval)	adjusted*	
Fish advice	0.71	(0.54 - 0.92)	0.71	p<0.05
Fat advice	0.97	(0.75 - 1.27)	1.00	
Fibre advice	1.23	(0.95 - 1.60)	1.27	

*adjusted for previous history, x-ray appearance and treatment

Table VI. Effects of dietary intervention on IHD events (Diet and Reinfarction Trial)

Dietary intervention	Risk ratio			Significance level
	unadjusted	(95% confidence interval)	adjusted*	
Fish advice	0.84	(0.67 - 1.07)	0.84	-
Fat advice	0.91	(0.71 - 1.15)	0.91	-
Fibre advice	1.21	(0.95 - 1.53)	1.23	-

*adjusted for previous history, x-ray appearance and treatment

which might have influenced the results. The group taking fatty fish showed a risk ratio of 0.71 compared with the other subjects (i.e. a reduction of 29% in deaths). The advice on fat or fibre was not associated with any reduction in mortality - indeed, mortality was non-significantly higher in subjects given fibre advice than in other subjects.

A similar analysis for IHD events (i.e. new myocardial infarcts plus deaths attributed to IHD) is shown in table VI. None of the three dietary interventions is significantly associated with the incidence of events.

Figure 1 shows the survival curves of the groups with a high and low intake of n-3 PUFA. The early divergence of the two curves suggests that an increased n-3

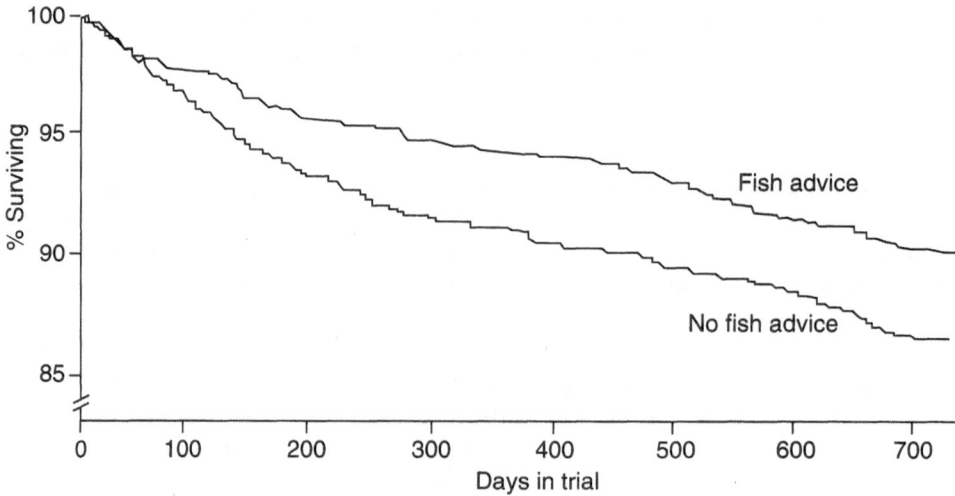

Fig. 1. Survival of two dietary groups in Diet and Reinfarction Trial.

PUFA intake rapidly confers some protection. This observation, combined with the lack of a significant effect on reinfarction, suggests that mechanisms may be operating other than a slowing of atherosclerosis or inhibition of thrombosis. In experimental animals, a raised intake of n-3 PUFA has been shown to protect against fatal arrhythmias occurring during myocardial ischaemia and reperfusion.[9] An anti-arrhythmic effect of n-3 PUFA in patients with IHD is therefore a possible explanation.

This hypothesis clearly needs further assessment in more specific investigations. Another controlled trial is currently testing the protective effect of fatty fish in patients with angina pectoris. Further studies are needed to show whether the protective effect of n-3 PUFA is mediated by a reduction of the electrical instability of the myocardium during acute infarction or by a decrease in the frequency and severity of episodes of ischaemia.

References

1. Kromhout D., Bosschieter E.B., Coulander C.deL.: The inverse relation between fish consumption and 20-year mortality from coronary heart disease. N. Engl. J. Med. 1985; 312: 1205-1209
2. Shekelle R.B., Missell L.V., Paul O., Shryock A.M., Stamler J.: Fish consumption and mortality from coronary heart disease. N Engl J Med 1985;313:820.
3. Dolecek T.A., Grandits G.: Dietary polyunsaturated fatty acids and mortality in the Multiple Risk Factor Intervention Trial (MRFIT). World Rev. Nutr. Diet. 1991; 66: 205-216
4. Vollset S.E., Heuch I., Bjelke E.: Fish consumption and mortality from coronary heart disease. N. Engl. J. Med. 1985; 313: 820-821
5. Curb J.D., Reed D.M.: Fish consumption and mortality from coronary heart disease. N. Engl. J. Med. 1985; 313: 821
6. Kristensen S.D., Schmidt E.B., Dyerberg J.: Dietary supplementation with n-3 polyunsaturated fatty acids and human platelet function: a review with particular emphasis on implications for cardiovascular disease. J. Internal Medicine 1989;225:141-150
7. Sanders T.A.B.: Influence of n-3 fatty acids on blood lipids. World Rev. Nutr. Diet 1991; 66: 358-366
8. Burr M.L., Fehily A.M., Gilbert J.F., Rogers S., Holliday R.M., Sweetnam P.M., Elwood P.C., Deadman N.M.: Effects of changes in fat, fish, and fibre intakes on death and myocardial reinfarction: Diet and Reinfarction Trial (DART). Lancet 1989; 2: 757-761
9. McLennan P.L., Abeywardena M.Y., Charnock J.S.: Reversal of the arrhythmogenic effects of long-term saturated fatty acid intake by dietary n-3 and n-6 polyunsaturated fatty acids. Am. J. Clin. Nutr. 1990; 51: 53-58

3. Modern Agriculture and Aquaculture and the n-6/n-3 Balance

A.P. SIMOPOULOS

The Center for Genetics, Nutrition and Health, Washington DC, USA

Introduction

Over the past 10 years, epidemiologic studies, animal studies and clinical investigations indicate that n-3 fatty acids are essential for normal growth and development of human beings. n-3 fatty acids are found in human milk whereas cow's milk does not contain n-3 fatty acids. n-3 fatty acids have hypolipidemic, antithrombotic and anti-inflammatory properties that contribute to the prevention and treatment of heart disease and hypertension. n-3 fatty acids, especially eicosapentaenoic acid (EPA) and docosahexaenoic acid (DHA) have beneficial effects in the treatment of a number of autoimmune diseases and disorders such as rheumatoid arthritis (and possibly lupus erythematosus), ulcerative colitis and psoriasis, and decrease the size and number of tumors in a variety of animal models. In epidemiologic studies, fish-eating populations have lower death rates from cardiovascular disease, except in situations where the saturated fat intake is high.[1-2]

It is considered that the current western diet is deficient in n-3 fatty acids in comparison with the diet during man's evolution, and that the enormously increased intake of n-6 fatty acids that has occurred since the turn of the century has contributed to the imbalance in the n-6/n-3 ratio.[3-7] This paper examines the status of the n-6/n-3 ratio in the Western diet and some of the causes that have led the n-6/n-3 imbalance.

Evolutionary Aspects

Modern human beings (*homo sapiens sapiens*) appeared about 40,000 years ago and the human genetic constitution has changed little since then. Hunter-gatherers consumed wild game (hunting, fishing) and wild vegetables. These are the foods that man is genetically "programmed" to eat, digest and metabolize. The development of agriculture began 10,000 years ago but even that had a minimal influence on our genes. The retention of intestinal lactase is the best example of man's genetic adaptability to nutrition. The new developments in food production and food processing over the past 150 years are too recent to influence our genetic constitution. Therefore, the diets available to humans prior to agricultural development are still the diets for which we are genetically programmed today. The foods that were available then varied widely in accordance with the paleontological period, the seasons of the year and the geographic location. Such a diet provided a variety of foods suitable for the omnivor which is characteristic of most primates. The differences between the diets of early humans and the diets of industrialized societies have been considered to have important implications for health.[1-4]

Information on the diet of early man is obtained from archaeological studies and from observations of present day hunter-gatherer societies. Based on estimates from studies in paleolithic nutrition and modern day hunter-gatherer populations, man evolved on a diet that was much lower in saturated fat than today's diet. Paleolithic diet had less total fat and more essential fatty acids and a much higher ratio of polyunsaturated fatty acids (PUFA)/saturates than ours. Our paleolithic ancestors consumed more structural and less depot fat.

Furthermore, the diet contained roughly equal amounts of n-6 and n-3 polyunsaturated fatty acids[3-6] (Fig. 1, Tab. I). Wild animals and birds who feed on wild

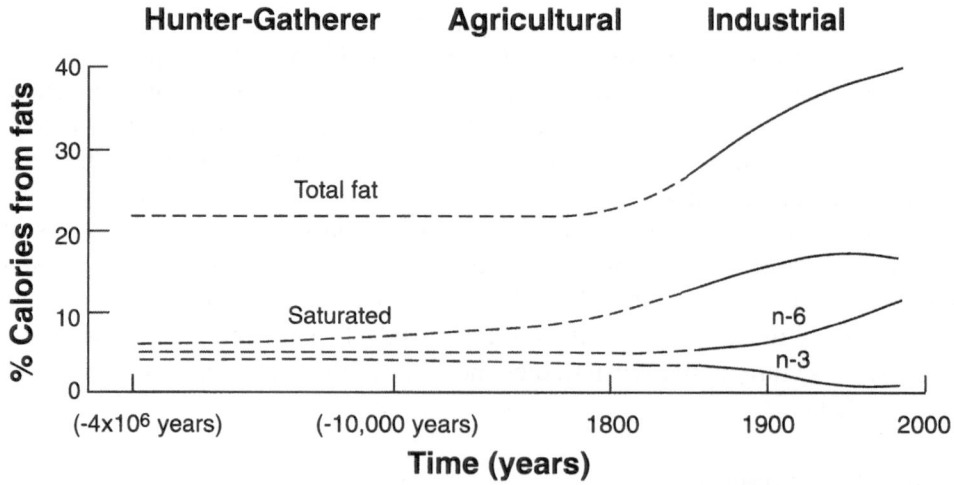

Fig. 1. Scheme of the relative percentages of different dietary fatty acids (saturated fatty acids and n-6 and n-3 unsaturated fatty acids) and possible changes subsequent to industrial food processing, involving fattening of animal husbandry and hydrogenation of fatty acids (Adapted from Leaf et al.[3]).

Table I. Characteristics of hunter-gatherer and Western lifestyles

Characteristic	Hunter-gatherer lifestyle	Western lifestyle
Physical Activity Level	*high*	*low*
Diet		
Energy-density	low	high
Energy intake	moderate	high
Protein	high	low-moderate
animal	high	low-moderate
vegetable	very low	low-moderate
Carbohydrate	low-moderate (slowly absorbed)	moderate (rapidly absorbed)
fiber	high	low
Fat	low	high
vegetable	very low	moderate to high
animal	low polyunsaturated	high saturated

plants are very lean with a carcass fat content of only 3.9%[7] and contain about five times more polyunsaturated fat per gram than is found in domestic livestock. Most importantly, 4% of the fat of wild animals contains EPA.

Food Production

Modern agriculture, with its emphasis on production, has decreased the n-3 fatty acid content in many foods: green leafy vegetables, animal meats, eggs and even fish.[8-10] Foods from edible wild plants contain a good balance of n-6 and n-3 fatty acids and are rich in vitamin C and carotenoids.[4] Wild purslane contains 10 times as much n-3 fatty acids as cultivated green vegetables such as lettuce and spinach[8] (Tab. II).

Modern aquaculture produces fish that contain less n-3 fatty acids than fish living naturally in the ocean, rivers and lakes.[10] In a study by van Vliet and Katan, the ratio of n-3 to n-6 fatty acids was significantly lower in cultured than in wild fish

Table II. Fatty acid content of plants.[8] (mg/g of wet weight)

Fatty Acid	Purslane	Spinach	Red Leaf Lettuce	Buttercrunch Lettuce	Mustard
14:0	0.16	0.03	0.03	0.01	0.02
16:0	0.81	0.16	0.10	0.07	0.13
18:0	0.20	0.01	0.01	0.02	0.02
18:1n-9	0.43	0.04	0.01	0.03	0.01
18:2n-6	0.89	0.14	0.12	0.10	0.12
18:3n-3	4.05	0.89	0.31	0.26	0.48
20:5n-3	0.01	0.00	0.00	0.00	0.00
22:6n-3	0.00	0.00	0.002	0.001	0.001
Other	1.95	0.43	0.12	0.11	0.32
Total fatty acid content	8.50	1.70	0.702	0.60	1.101

(2 vs 5 in eel, 2 vs 7 in trout, and 6 vs 11 in salmon).[10] Cultured fish contained less n-3 fatty acids, more n-6 fatty acids and more total fat than fish in the wild (Tab. III).

In another study, Simopoulos and Salem found that the ratio of n-6 to n-3 fatty acids was 1.3 in the Greek egg from free-ranging chickens versus 19.4 in the supermarket egg[9] (Tab. IV). With its emphasis on increased production, industrialization has led to the development of a chicken feed that promotes increased egg production because it contains higher levels of protein, amino acids, and linoleic acid. These dietary components are reflected in the composition of the supermarket eggs consumed today: they are high in n-6 and low in n-3 fatty acids. In addition, modern agriculture, with the emphasis on grain feeds for domestic livestock, led to further increases in saturated fat and n-6 fatty acids (grains are rich in n-6 fatty acids).

The increased consumption of n-6 acids in the last 100 years is due to a large extent to the development of technology at the turn of the century that marked the beginning of the modern vegetable oil industry (Fig. 1). Furthermore, prior to the 1940's, cod liver oil was ingested mainly by children as a source of vitamins A and D, with the usual dose being "a teaspoon". Once these vitamins were synthesized, consumption of cod liver oil was drastically decreased, and there was a decrease in the consumption of fish.

Table III. Fat content and fatty acid composition of wild and cultured trout, eel, and salmon°

	Trout (Salmo gairdneri and Salmo trutta fario)		Eel (Anguilla anguilla)		Salmon (Salmo salar)	
	Wild (*n = 2*)	*Cultured* (*n = 9*)	*Wild* (*n = 4*)	*Cultured* (*n = 4*)	*Wild* (*n = 2*)	*Cultured* (*n = 2*)
Fat (g/100g)	5±3	6 ±1	21±6	30 ±2 *	10 ±0.1	16±0.6**
Fatty acids (g/100 g fatty acid)						
18:3 n-3	3±2	1 ±0.3**	2±2	1 ±0.3	1 ±0.1	1 ±0.1
20:5 n-3	7±0.6	4 ±1 **	4±2	3 ±0.6	5 ±0.2	5 ±0.1
22:6 n-3	15±2	13 ±1 *	4±2	6 ±0.4	10 ±2	7 ±0.1*
Other n-3***	5±0.6	2 ±0.7**	3±1	2 ±0.2*	3 ±0.5	4 ±0.1
18:2 n-6	4±3	9 ±2 **	2±2	5 ±0.3**	1 ±0.1	3 ±0.1
Other n-6****	1±0.4	0.6±0.1**	2±0.3	0.4±0.1**	0.2±0.1	0.5±0.1
Sum of n-3	30±0.2	20 ±3 **	14±3	12 ±1	20 ±2	17 ±0.2
Sum of n-6	5±3	9 ±2 *	3±1	6 ±0.3**	2 ±0.1	3 ±0.1**
n-3 : n-6	7±5	2 ±0.6**	5±2	2 ±0.3	11 ±2	6 ±0.1*

Reproduced from van Vliet T, Katan MB[10]

° x ± SD, n, number of lots; each lot consisted of about six trout or eel or one or two salmon

* p<0.05 compared with wild fish; **p<0.01 compared with wild fish;

*** 18:4 n-3 + 20:3 n-3 + 22:5 n-3; ****20:4 n-6 + 22:4 n-6.

In the United States, recent studies by the Department of Agriculture indicate that the n-3 fatty acids levels per capita per day in 1985 were 46 mg of EPA, 78 mg for DHA and 2.8 g of LNA.

The percentage contribution of EPA and DHA was 4 percent, whereas that of LNA was 96 percent. Of interest is the fact that paleolithic nutrition contained more EPA and DHA and less LNA than today's diet.

Conclusions and Recommendations

Thus, an absolute and relative change of n-6 and n-3 fatty acids in the food supply of western societies has occurred over the last 100 years with an estimated ratio of n-6/n-3 of about 20-30/1 rather than the 2-5-7/1 found in human milk or 1/1 estimated from paleolithic nutrition. Many dietary studies and interventions have been carried out and dietary recommendations have been made in relation to saturated fat and cholesterol.

20

Table IV. Fatty acid levels in chicken egg yolks*

Fatty Acid	Greek Egg	Supermarket Egg
*mg of fatty acid***		
Saturated fats		
14:0	1.10	0.70
15:0	-	0.07
16:0	77.60	56.66
17:0	0.66	0.34
18:0	21.30	22.88
Total	*100.66*	*80.65*
Monounsaturated fats		
16:1n-7	21.70	4.67
18:1	120.50	109.97
20:1n-9	0.58	0.68
22:1n-9	-	-
24:1n-9	-	0.04
Total	*142.78*	*115.36*
n-6 Fatty acids		
18:2n-6	16.00	26.14
18:3n-6	-	0.25
20:2n-6	0.17	0.36
20:3n-6	0.46	0.47
20:4n-6	5.40	5.02
22:4n-6	0.70	0.37
22:5n-6	0.29	1.20
Total	*23.02*	*33.81*
n-3 Fatty acids		
18:3n-3	6.90	0.52
20:3n-3	0.16	0.03
20:5n-3	1.20	-
22:5n-3	2.80	0.09
22:6n-3	6.60	1.09
Total	*17.66*	*1.73*
Ratio of n-6 to n-3	1.3	19.4
Ratio of fatty acids to saturated fats	0.4	0.44

* The eggs were hard-boiled, and their fatty acid composition and lipid content were assessed as described elsewhere; ** Per gram of egg yolk.

The indiscriminate recommendation to replace saturated fats with PUFAs from vegetable oils has led to increased amounts of n-6 fatty acids in man's diet over the past 50-60 years.

Thus, man has been exposed to pharmacologic doses of n-6 fatty acids for the first time in his evolution.

Since the fatty acid composition of cell membranes modulates important cell functions, yet the fatty acids in the membrane are dependent on dietary intake, it is obvious that in referring to PUFAs it is essential to distinguish between n-3 and n-6 fatty acids in making dietary recommendations.

Simply using the ratio of polyunsaturates to saturates (P/S) is inappropriate and inadequate, based on the knowledge we have today. However, the amount of n-3 fatty acids in the diet and their effects on health and disease have not been considered in the development of dietary guidelines by national governments except for the most recent Canadian Nutrition Recommendations. In view of the fact that n-3 fatty acids have different metabolic effects than those of the n-6 series and that n-3 fatty acids are essential for normal growth and development and for overall health, accurate knowledge of the amount and type of n-3 fatty acids in foods is essential. Both terrestrial and marine sources of n-3 fatty acids are important in this regard.

Differences also exist among the saturated fatty acids, lauric, myristic, palmitic, and stearic, and between the *cis* and *trans* forms of fatty acids in terms of their atherogenic and thrombogenic properties.

In making dietary recommendations, the importance of considering the function of the different types of fatty acids (n-3, n-6, n-9 and the various saturated fatty acids) rather than simply total fat (percentage of calories from fat) or the amount of polyunsaturates, is now being accepted. Fatty acids should be considered:

1. in terms of their overall metabolic effects in growth and development;
2. for their effects on serum lipids, inflammation, thrombus formation, and tumor development.

Polyunsaturated fatty acids (n-6 and n-3) should contribute 10% of calories with equal amounts of n-6 and n-3 fatty acids.

In order to improve the n-6/n-3 imbalance it will be necessary to decrease consumption of n-6 fatty acids while increasing the consumption of n-3 fatty acids, particularly eicosapentaenoic acid and docosahexaenoic acid. This can be accomplished by increasing the amount of fish in the diet to 2-3 times per week, or taking 1 g of fish oils per day.

References

1. Simopoulos A.P.: Omega-3 fatty acids in health and disease and in growth and development. Am. J. Clin. Nutr. 1991; 54: 438-463
2. Simopoulos A.P., Kifer R.R., Martin R.E., Barlow S.M.: Health Effects of ω3 Polyunsaturated Fatty Acids in Seafoods.World Rev. Nutr. Diet, Basel: Karger, 1991; vol. 66
3. Leaf A., Weber P.C.: A new era for science in nutrition. Am. J. Clin. Nutr. 1987; 45 (supplement): 1048-1053
4. Simopoulos A.P.: Terrestrial sources of omega-3 fatty acids: purslane. In: Quebedeaux B, Bliss F., (Eds.) *Horticulture and Human Health: Contributions of Fruits and Vegetables.* Englewood Cliffs, N.J.: Prentice-Hall 1988; 93-107
5. Eaton S.B., Konner M.: Paleolithic nutrition. A consideration of its nature and current implications. N. Engl. J. Med. 1985; 312: 283-289
6. Simopoulos A.P.: Genetics and nutrition: Or what your genes can tell you about nutrition. In: Simopoulos A.P., Childs B. (Eds.): *Genetic Variation and Nutrition.* World Rev. Nutr. Diet, Basel: Karger 1990; vol. 63: 25-34
7. Crawford M.A.: Fatty acid ratios in free-living and domestic animals. Lancet 1968; 1: 1239-1333
8. Simopoulos A.P., Salem Jr. N.: Purslane: A terrestrial source of omega-3 fatty acids. N. Engl. J. Med. 1986; 315: 833
9. Simopoulos A.P., Salem Jr. N.: n-3 fatty acids in eggs from range-fed Greek chickens. N. Engl. J. Med. 1989; 321: 1412
10. van Vliet T., Katan M.B.: Lower ratio of n-3 to n-6 fatty acids in cultured than in wild fish. Am. J. Clin. Nutr. 1990; 51: 1-2

4. Fish Consumption and Blood Pressure: Epidemiological Data

S.D. KRISTENSEN
University Department of Cardiology, Skejby Hospital, Aarhus N, Denmark

Two recent controlled studies have shown that dietary supplementation with n-3 polyunsaturated fatty acids (PUFA) causes a decrease in blood pressure in patients with mild hypertension.[1,2] The purpose of this paper is to review the epidemiological data on the relation between fish intake and blood pressure.

The evidence arises from three different lines of research:

1. studies on blood pressure values in Eskimos;
2. comparisons of blood pressure values in subjects with different intake of fatty acids in other communities;
3. analysis of the relationship between blood pressure and content of n-3 PUFA in cell membranes.

Studies in Eskimos

The first large study on blood pressure measurements in Eskimos was published by Ehrstrom in 1951.[3] He studied 1071 subjects living in the Umanak district in North Greenland and compared blood pressure values to a Finnish control group (857 subjects). The control group was not matched for age and sex. No information on the dietary habits of the subjects studied was available. However, it is likely that the Eskimos had a very high intake of n-3 PUFA. The author concluded that for subjects younger than 30 years old no difference in systolic blood pressure was found, whereas for subjects older than 30 years higher systolic blood pressure values were found in the Eskimos. Although the data on diastolic blood pressure values were not given in the paper, the author states in his conclusion, that diastolic hypertension (>110 mmHg) was rare in the Eskimos.

Scott and coworkers measured blood pressure in the sitting position in 842 Eskimo men and reported that blood pressure values were not different from values obtained in an age- and sex-matched American control group.[4] In the Eskimos a weak correlation between mean blood pressure and age was found. The Eskimos were all members of the Alaskan National Guard and no information on their diet was given in the paper.

In another study blood pressure was measured in the supine position in 177 Eskimos at the time of admission to the hospital in Thule, Greenland.[5] Blood pressure was found to be unrelated to age in the Eskimos. When compared to a Danish control group with approximately the same age- and sex-distribution, the incidence of hypertension was lower in the Eskimos. However, the Danish controls were out-patients examined by general practitioners, and it is likely that differences in body posture and in the frequency of acute illness may in part explain the reported difference in blood pressure.

In a study performed on two Eskimo groups comprising 158 and 252 subjects, where blood pressure measurements were more carefully standardized, Bjerager et al.[6] were able to demonstrate a significant increase in blood pressure with age. The blood pressure values in the Eskimos in this study were not different from values obtained in an age- and sex-matched Danish control group.

Finally, Jørgensen et al.[7] measured blood pressure in 20 Greenland Eskimos with a documented high intake of n-3 PUFA and were unable to demonstrate any difference in blood pressure when compared to age-and sex-matched Danish controls. In the same study plasma renin levels were found to be higher in Eskimos, whereas no difference in urinary sodium excretion was found.

In conclusion, the knowledge we can obtain from studies in Eskimos does not support the hypothesis that a high intake of n-3 PUFA causes any change in blood pressure.

Blood Pressure and Fish Intake in other Populations

In Taiwan, where cardiovascular disease is an important problem, Tseng[8] compared the blood pressure in 5,585 subjects living in a fishing area to a group of 14,304 subjects living in an agricultural area. The group were well-matched for age and sex.

The blood pressure recordings were performed in the sitting position by 15 different physicians. Both systolic and diastolic blood pressure and also the incidence of hypertension were significantly higher in the group living in the fishing area. Only very little information on the dietary differences in the two groups is available. The intake of salt was probably higher in the fishing population and the author suggests this may account for the increase in blood pressure in this group.

Kagawa et al.[9] studied a group of Japanese subjects (n=77, age > 65 years) living on a fishing island and compared blood pressure values to a group of age- and sex-matched Japanese. The group from the fishing island had higher serum eicosapentaenoic acid (n-3 20:5) levels and lower blood pressure values than the control group. Also the incidence of hypertension was lower in the group with a high intake of fish. However, the group living on the fishing island had a lower salt intake than the control group.

Robinson and Day[10] measured the blood pressure in two groups of East African tribesmen. The diastolic blood pressure was significantly higher in the group of fish-eaters (n=22), when compared to the group of non-fish-eaters (n=45). Detailed information on the composition of the diets in the two groups is lacking, and the difference in blood pressure between the two groups may well be due to other factors than the intake of fish.

In a study conducted in Northern Norway two age- and sex-matched groups of males (n=14 in both groups) were studied.[11] The group living in the coastal area had a higher intake of fish. However, there was no significant difference in the content of n-3 PUFA in the platelet membranes nor in blood pressure between the two groups.

Finally, in the Zutphen study, where the dietary intake of fish was estimated on the basis of interviews, the blood pressure in the 852 middle-aged Dutch males included in the study was not correlated to the consumption of fish.[12] A similar conclusion was reached in a Swedish study comprising 1,462 women.[13]

The Relation between Content of n-3 PUFA in Cell Membranes or Serum Lipids and Blood Pressure

Miettinen et al. studied the fatty acid composition of serum lipids in patients with ischaemic heart disease and in healthy Finnish male controls.[14] In the controls the content of eicosapentaenoic acid (n-3 20:5) was found to be inversely correlated to blood pressure. Wood and co-workers[15] measured the fatty acid composition of adipose tissue and platelet membranes in Scottish males with and without ischaemic heart disease. No correlation between the content of n-3 PUFA and blood pressure values could be demonstrated.

In a study from Southern Italy the fatty acid composition of adipose tissue and the blood pressure was measured in 74 healthy, middle-aged men.[16] When the subjects were divided into quintiles according to their diastolic blood pressure, the subjects with high diastolic blood pressure had a significantly higher amount of eicosapentaenoic acid (n-3 20:5) in their adipose tissue than the group with low blood pressure. Surprisingly, when the same persons were interviewed on their dietary habits, the group with high diastolic blood pressure had a significantly lower intake of fish than the group with low diastolic blood pressure.

26

Conclusion

As stated above most of the studies investigating whether a high dietary intake of fish is associated with a lowering of blood pressure suffer from methodological limitations. In particular the amount of fish consumed may have been too low in many of the studies. Also, lack of standardization of blood pressure measurement and poorly defined control groups may hamper the data.

However, in conclusion, there is not much epidemiological evidence that dietary fish intake has any major effect on blood pressure.

References

1. Knapp H.R., FitzGerald G.A.: The antihypertensive effects of fish oil: a controlled study of polyunsaturated fatty acid supplements in essential hypertension. N. Engl. J. Med. 1989; 320: 1037-1043
2. Bønaa K.H., Bjerve K.S., Straume B., Gram T.T., Thelle D.: Effect of eicosapentaenoic and docosahexaenoic acids on blood pressure in hypertension. A population-based intervention trial from the Tromsø study. N. Engl. J. Med. 1990; 322: 795-801
3. Ehrstrom M.C.: Medical studies in North Greenland 1948-9. Blood pressure, hypertension and arteriosclerosis in relation to food and mode of living. Acta Med. Scand. 1951; 160: 416-422
4. Scott E.M., Griffith I.V., Hoskins D.D., Whaley R.D.: Serum-cholesterol levels and blood-pressure of Alaskan Eskimo men. Lancet 1958; 2: 667-668
5. Simper L.B.: Blodtrykket hos polareskimoer. Ugeskrift for laeger, 1976; 138: 1757-1758
6. Bjerager P., Kromann N., Thygesen K., Haravald B.: Blodtryk hos gronlandere. Ugeskrift for laeger 1980; 142: 2278-2280
7. Jørgensen K.A., Nielsen A.H., Dyerberg J.: Haemostatic factors and renin in Greenland Eskimos on a high eicosapentaenoic acid intake. Acta Med. Scand. 1986; 219: 473-479
8. Tseng W-P.: Blood pressure and hypertension in an agricultural and a fishing population in Taiwan. Amer. J. Epidemiol. 1967; 86: 513-525
9. Kagawa Y., Nishizawa M., Suzuki M., et al.: Eicosapolyenoic acids of serum lipids of Japanese islanders with low incidence of cardiovascular disease. J. Nutr. Sci. Vitaminol. 1982; 28: 441-453
10. Robinson D., Day J.: Low plasma triglyceride levels in lake dwelling East African tribesmen - a fishy story? Int. J. Epidemiol. 1986; 15: 183-187
11. Simonson T., Vartun A., Lyngmo V., Nordøy A.: Coronary heart disease, serum lipids, platelets and dietary fish in two communities in Northern Norway. Acta Med. Scand. 1987; 222: 237-245
12. Kromhout D., Bosschieter E.B., Coulander C.D.L.: The inverse relation between fish consumption and 20-year mortality from coronary heart disease. N. Engl. J. Med. 1985; 312: 1205-1209
13. Lapidus L., Andersson H., Bengtsson C., Bosaeus I.: Dietary habits in relation to incidence of cardiovascular disease and death in women: a 12-year follow-up of participants in the population study of women in Gothenburg, Sweden. Am. J. Clin. Nutr. 1986; 44: 444-448
14. Miettinen T.A., Naukkarinen V., Huttunen J.K., Mattila S., Kumlin T.: Fatty-acid composition of serum lipids predicts myocardial infarction. Br. J. Med. 1982; 285: 993-996
15. Wood D.A., Riemersma R.A., Butler S. et al.: Linoleic and eicosapentaenoic acids in adipose tissue and platelets and risk of coronary heart disease. Lancet 1987; i: 177-183
16. Rubba P., Mancini M., Fidanza F., et al.: Adipose tissue fatty acids and blood pressure in middle-aged men from Southern Italy. Int. J. Epidemiol. 1987; 16: 528-531

5. The Effect of n-3 Fatty Acids on Cardiovascular Risk Factors: An Overview

A. NORDØY

Department of Medicine, Tromsø University Hospital, Tromsø, Norway

Risk Factors and Coronary Heart Disease

It is well established that it is possible to evaluate the probability of a severe cardiovascular event, such as an acute myocardial infarction or a stroke, by assessing the presence or absence of the so-called risk factors. Some of these risk factors are well defined; however, others have emerged from analysis of more recent epidemiological studies and from a better understanding of the biochemical and pathophysiological mechanisms leading to atherosclerosis and thrombosis. These new risk factors may in the near future be very helpful in identifying subjects at high risk and in evaluating the beneficial effect of interventions.

Several studies, and among them the Framingham study, have identified and characterized the importance of age, sex and genetic factors in influencing the risk of a cardiovascular event.

Also, the role of smoking, elevated blood pressure, dyslipidaemia and blood hypercoagulability has been verified and quantitated. Unlike the first group of coronary risk factors, these factors can be altered by modification of life-style, including dietary habits of each individual, and by the use of pharmacological treatments.

The Effect of n-3 Fatty Acids on Lipids and Haemostasis

In the analysis of the possible role of n-3 fatty acids in reducing cardiovascular risk, it seems useful to evaluate the effect of these fatty acids on both the well established risk factors and on the less documented risk factors.

28

In order to quantitate the effect of an increased intake of n-3 fatty acids on some of these risk factors, a study with a total duration of 24 weeks was recently performed (Fig. 1).[1]

In this study, after a run-in period during which the participants were on their usual diet, they underwent, for three weeks, a diet rich in fats (40 % of the total caloric intake) represented by saturated fatty acids for about 20 % of the total caloric intake. Then the subjects were on a similar diet, but with the addition of n-3 fatty acids (n-3 fatty acids representing 2 % of the total intake of calories); and then they returned to their usual diet for nine weeks. Patients were then put on a diet relatively poor in lipids (25 % of the total caloric intake with saturated fatty acids accounting for 10 % of the total caloric intake), and finally put on a similar diet but with the addition of n-3 fatty acids (n-3 fatty acids representing 2 % of the total intake of calories).

The results of the study showed first of all that the addition of relatively modest amounts of n-3 fatty acids was indeed associated with an increase in the serum content of these fatty acids, indicating the possibility of modulating the phospholipid composition

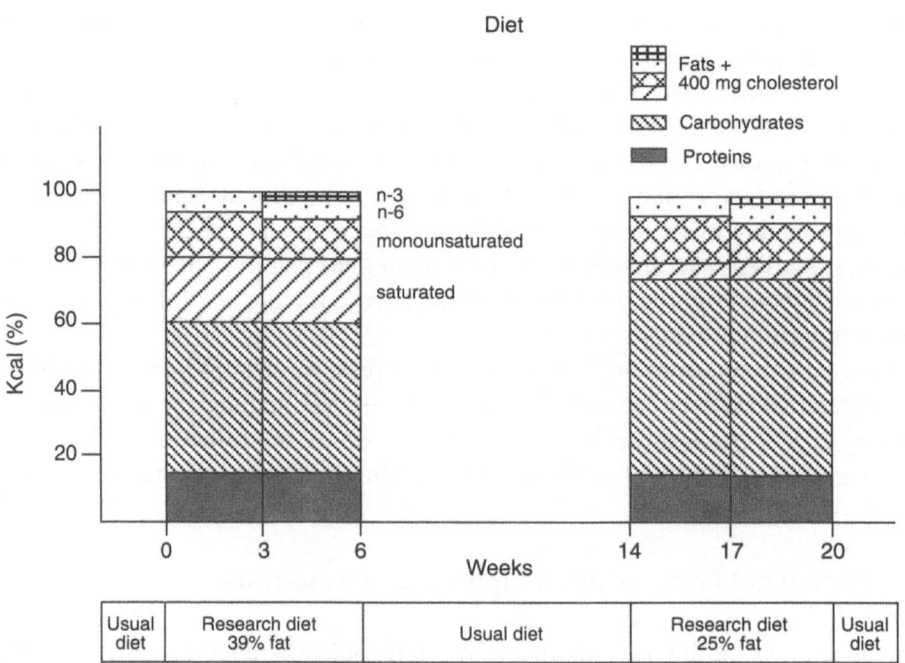

Fig. 1. Design of the study presented (see text for further details).

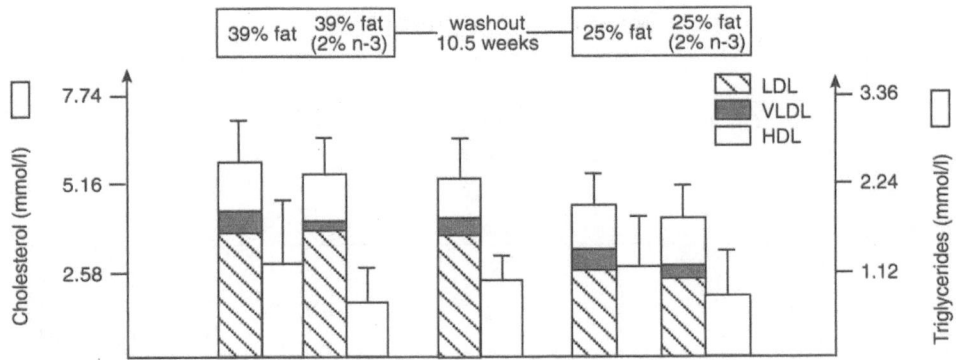

Fig. 2. The effect of various diets on plasma lipids. Results are means with standard deviations.

of cytoplasmic membranes by modifying the diet. Analysis of changes in risk factors focused on two specific aspects: lipids and haemostasis. Plasma lipid profile showed some important changes throughout the study, as illustrated in figure 2.

The addition of n-3 fatty acids to the diet thus resulted in a significant reduction in VLDL-cholesterol and in triglycerides both during the fat-enriched and the fat-deprived diets. HDL-cholesterol and LDL-cholesterol on the other hand were not significantly altered. A reduction in total cholesterol levels was observed when values measured during the diet poor in fats were compared to those obtained during the diet rich in fats. In contrast, levels of apolipoproteins were not modified by any dietetic regimen, suggesting that the metabolism of the protein component of lipoproteins was not altered by these short-term changes of the dietary n-3 fatty acids.

The data on the effect of n-3 fatty acids on plasma lipids are in agreement with those obtained in other studies. Indeed, as summarized by Harris in a recent review,[3] the most evident effect of n-3 fatty acids is to reduce triglyceride levels.

This effect is most pronounced in patients with isolated hypertriglyceridaemia and in this population sometimes associated with an increase in LDL-cholesterol (Fig. 3).

It is also of interest to note anecdotal reports of patients with severe hypertriglyceridaemia associated with recurrent episodes of acute pancreatitis in which treatment with n-3 fatty acids markedly reduced triglyceride levels and prevented further episodes of acute pancreatitis (Fig. 4).[9]

However, the quantitation of this effect of n-3 fatty acids will require clinical trials targeted to answer this problem.

Levels of several coagulation factors such as factor VII, fibrinogen and antithrombin III were not significantly modified by any of the dietary regimens.

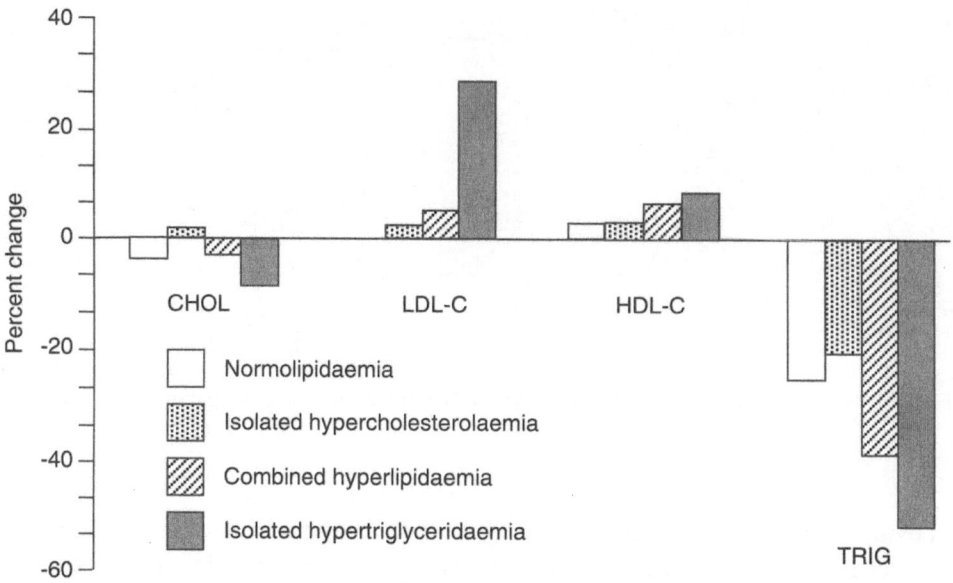

Fig. 3. The effect of n-3 fatty acids on plasma lipids in normolipidaemic subjects and in patients with hyperlipidaemia. The percent changes from baseline are shown.[3]

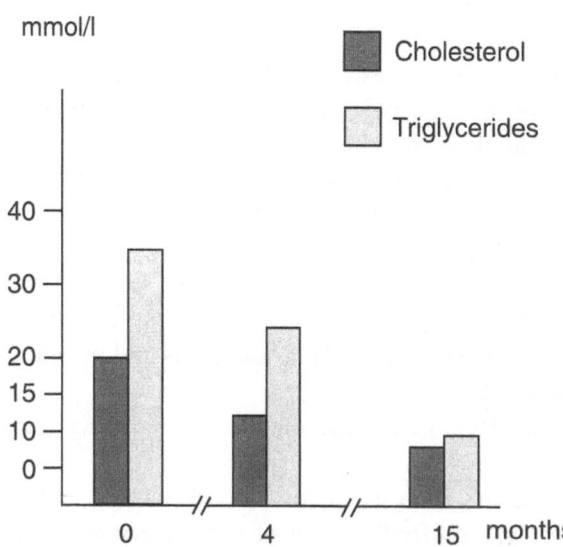

Fig. 4. The effect of n-3 fatty acids given as daily fish meals and 30 ml cod liver oil on serum lipids in a patient with combined hyperlipidaemia.[9]

However, interesting data were observed for bleeding time, a parameter reflecting platelet function, and possibly related to thrombotic tendency.

In fact, the simple addition of n-3 fatty acids to a diet rich in saturated fats did not modify bleeding time, whereas the combination of a diet poor in saturated fats and rich in n-3 fatty acids was associated with a significant increase in bleeding time, suggesting a reduced tendency to thrombosis. This observation implies that probably in platelets saturated fatty acids and n-3 fatty acids might antagonize each other so that the beneficial effect of the latter is evident only when the negative effect of saturated fatty acids is removed.

Analysis of the data on urinary excretion of prostaglandins and thromboxanes showed a reduction in both types of metabolites after ingestion of n-3 fatty acids during both the diet rich in saturated fat (diet 2) and the diet low in saturated fat (diet 5).

Overall, data obtained in this study indicate that an increased intake of n-3 fatty acids induces a favourable change in some risk factors, such as in lipid profile and in the tendency to thrombosis as well as in eicosanoid metabolism.

Other Effects of n-3 Fatty Acids in Relation to Coronary Heart Disease

It is of importance that the abovementioned effects of dietary n-3 fatty acids on lipid pattern and haemostasis are associated with a reduction in blood pressure, which is another important risk factor for cardiovascular disease.[4]

Likely to be even more important, however, are the effect of n-3 fatty acids on cellular reactivity.

For example, we have previously evaluated the effect of n-3 fatty acids on endothelial cell function by measuring the synthesis of tissue thromboplastin after stimulation with lipopolysaccharides (Fig. 5).[5]

The data indicated that n-3 fatty acids decreased thromboplastin activity. n-3 fatty acids may also modulate the cellular response to several pro-inflammatory stimuli not only in endothelial cells but also in platelets, monocytes and granulocytes, as recently reviewed.[6]

Finally, it is possible that n-3 fatty acids may have a direct effect on cardiac myocytes.

In fact, alteration in the content of cardiac membrane phospholipids has important consequences for ionic transport responsible for cellular excitability, on receptor responsiveness, for the susceptibility to peroxidation during ischaemia and reperfusion, and for electrical stability.[7,8]

All these factors may potentially reduce cardiac susceptibility to malignant ventricular arrhytmias.

32

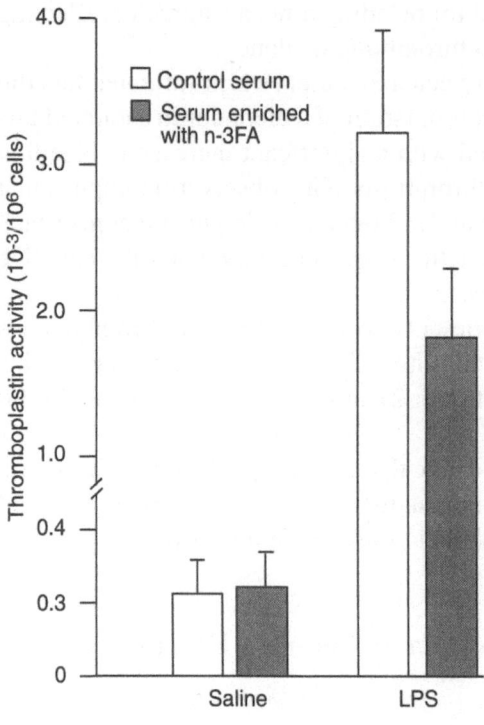

Fig. 5. The effect of n-3 fatty acids on tissue thromboplastin production from endothelial cells in unstimulated conditions (saline) and when stimulated with lipopolysaccharide (LPS).

Table I. Traditional risk factors for coronary heart disease and n-3 fatty acids

1. Serum lipids:

        Total Cholesterol ↑
        LDL   Cholesterol ↑
        HDL   Cholesterol ↓
        VLDL Cholesterol ↓   Triglycerides ↓ ↓

2. Smoking
3. Family - CHD
4. CHD or other atherosclerotic disease
5. Hypertension ↓
6. Diabetes
7. Dietary saturated fatty acids and cholesterol ↓
8. Age and sex
9. Coagulation/fibrinolysis: AT-III?
                              VII ↓
                              t-PA/PAI?
                              Fibrinogen?

Table II. Cellular processes, n-3 fatty acids and coronary heart disease.

---

1. Blood cells

Platelets: ↑ EPA/DHA, ↓ AA, ↓ TXA$_2$, ↑ TXA$_3$
   ↓ Platelet aggregation and thrombosis
   ↓ Coronary constriction and vascular spasm

Monocytes/granulocytes:
   ↑ EPA/DHA, ↓ AA, ↓ Leukotrienes
   ↓ Coronary constriction
   ↓ Improved microcirculation
   ↓ Oxygen radicals and cellular damage
   ↓ Thromboplastin synthesis

2. Coronary arteries

Endothelial cells: ↑ EPA/DHA, ↓ AA, ↑ ↓ PGI$_2$
   ↑ Coronary vasodilatation
   ↓ Thromboplastin

3. Heart muscle

Myocytes: ↑ ↑ DHA, ↑ EPA, ↓ AA, ↓ LA

Membrane phospholipids in relation to:
a. Ion transport
b. Heart rate
c. Receptor
d. Stability
e. Peroxidation

Conclusion

In summary, n-3 fatty acids are indeed able to modify some of the well-known risk factors for cardiovascular disease (Tab. I) and are able to modulate the cellular response to several atherogenic stimuli (Tab. II). Ongoing and future studies are however needed to document the clinical relevance of these effects of n-3 fatty acids.

References

1. Nordøy A., Hatcher L., Connor W.E., Ullmann D.O.: The interaction of dietary saturated fat and fish oil upon the plasma lipids and lipoproteins in normal men. Submitted 1991

34

2. Nordøy A., Connor W.E., Goodnight Jr.S.: Do dietary fatty acids counteract the antithrombotic effects of n-3 fatty acids? Abstr. Tenth Inter. Symp. on Drugs Affecting Lipid Metabolism, Houston, Texas Nov. 8-11, 1989 p. 38

3. Harris WS.: Fish oils and plasma lipid and lipoprotein metabolism in humans: a critical review. J. Lipid Res. 1989; 30: 785-807

4. Bønaa K., Bjerve K.S., Straume B., Gran I.T., Thelle D.: Effect of eicosapentaenoic acids on blood pressure in hypertension. N. Engl. J. Med. 1990; 322: 795-801

5. Hansen J.B., Svensson B., Wilsgard L., Østerud B.: Serum enriched with n-3 polyunsaturated fatty acids inhibits procoagulant activity in endothelial cells. Blood Coagulation Fibrinolysis. 1991; 2: 515-519

6. Leaf A., Weber P.C.: Cardiovascular effects of n-3 fatty acids. N. Engl. J. Med. 1988; 318: 549-557

7. Nestel P.J.: Review: Fish oil and cardiac function. World Rev. Nutr. Diet. 1991; 66: 268-277

8. Charnock J.S.: Antiarrhythmic effects of fish oils. World Rev. Nutr. Diet. 1991; 66: 278-291

9. Onkiehong M., Nordøy A.: Fisk, tran og hyperlipemi. Tidsskr Nor Lægeforen 11: 1986; 912-913

6. n-3 Fatty Acids: Incorporation into Tissue Lipids and Interactions with Dietary Components

C. GALLI, E. TREMOLI, C. SIRTORI

Institute of Pharmacological Sciences and E. Grossi Paoletti Center, University of Milan, Italy

Digestion and absorption of n-3 fatty acids involve three different steps, namely their hydrolysis from the alcohol to which they are bound, their absorption, and their subsequent uptake and incorporation into membranes of various cell types. Gastrointestinal hydrolysis of lipids introduced with the diet and intestinal absorption of fatty acids are usually considered relatively simple processes for the human organism. However the absorption of lipids containing n-3 fatty acids presents some problems, related to the poor activity of pancreatic lipase towards these compounds.[1,2] Two preparations of n-3 fatty acids are nowadays commercially available: in one case eicosapentaenoic acid (EPA) and docosahexaenoic acid (DHA) are esterified in the form of triglycerides; in the other, they are bound to ethanol in the form of ethyl esters.

Generally, the absorption of ethyl esters is slower, their hydrolysis being less effective.[3] The administration of n-3 fatty acids in the form of ethyl esters, however, allows a reduction of total lipids administered to the patient, with the consequence of a better compliance during long-term treatment; another advantage of ethyl esters is that one can avoid the administration of other lipidic compounds (sterols, other fatty acids, lipid soluble contaminants) which may be present in conventional fish oil preparations.

In the present paper we will briefly review data obtained in a series of studies by our group, in which n-3 fatty acids have been administered to normolipidemic and hyperlipidemic subjects in the form of ethyl esters.

In a first series of studies 2.8 g of EPA and 1.7 g of DHA (in the form of 6 capsules per day of an ethyl ester preparation [K-85, Norsk Hydro, Norway] of fish oil) were administered for 6 weeks to 5 male normolipidemic volunteers. The incorporation of n-3 fatty acids into plasma lipids, lipoproteins and cell membranes of various cell types, such as platelets, polymorphonuclear leukocytes (PMN) and monocytes, were monitored. Also, the effects on plasma lipids and lipoproteins were monitored. Such a regimen in healthy volunteers did not induce significant variations in total cholesterol, triglycerides and the various lipid fractions (cholesterol, free cholesterol, triglycerides, phospholipids) of either HDL, VLDL or LDL. Measurement of baseline content of EPA and DHA in the different cell types revealed a different and unique composition for each cell type, with monocytes, as an example, having a higher baseline content of EPA (20:5) as compared to platelets and PMN (Figs. 1-3). After administration of n-3 fatty acids an increase in the content of EPA and DHA in all cell types was observed (Figs. 1-3). The degree of relative incorporation,

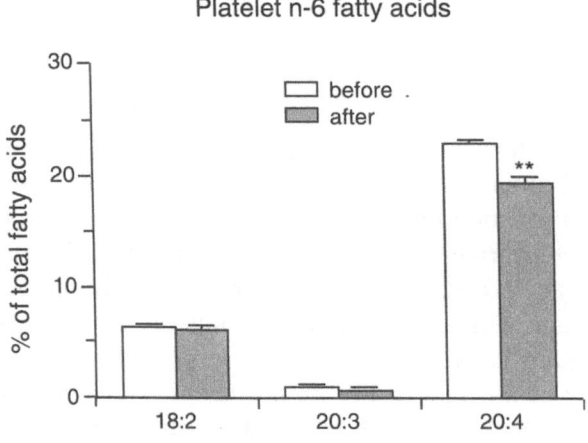

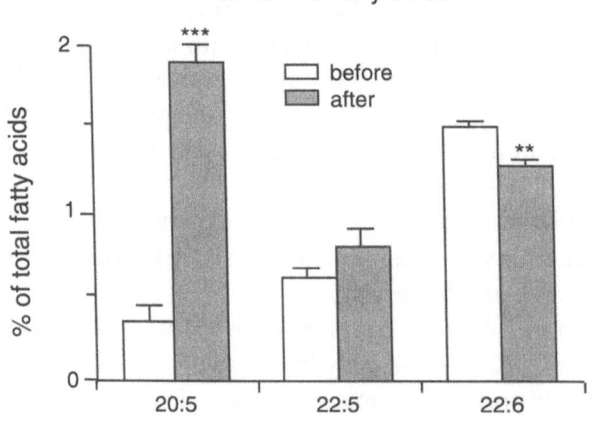

Fig. 1. Incorporation of n-6 (upper panel) and n-3 (lower panel) fatty acids as percent of total fatty acids, in platelet phospholipids of normolipidemic subjects before and after treatment. There were significant differences from corresponding values before treatment, at the following levels: **p<0.02; ***p<0.001.

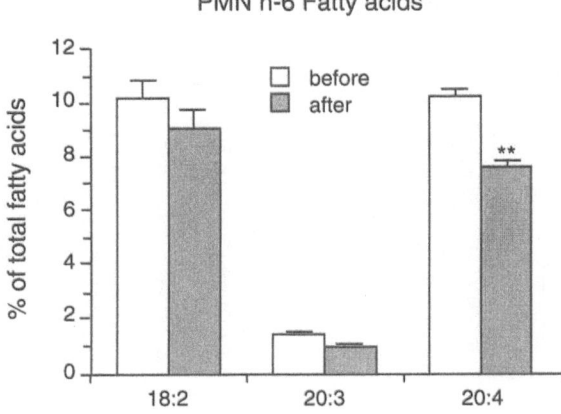

PMN n-6 Fatty acids

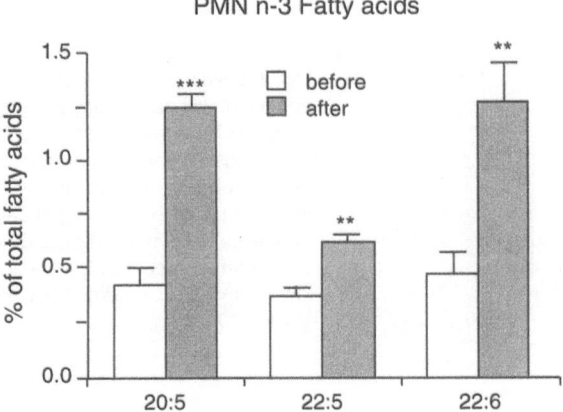

PMN n-3 Fatty acids

Fig. 2. Levels of n-6 (upper panel) and n-3 (lower panel) fatty acids, as percent of total fatty acids in polymorphonuclear leukocytes (PMN) phospholipids of normolipidemic subjects, before and after treatment. There were significant differences from corresponding values before treatment, at the following levels: **p<0.02; ***p<0.001.

however, was again different from cell to cell (Tab. I). These data suggest that the uptake and incorporation of n-3 fatty acids in cell membranes varies according to cell type; in particular, the EPA/DHA ratio varies quite markedly, probably due to the presence of a partial conversion of EPA to DHA or of some degree of retroconversion, all of which are probably specific for each cell type.

Similar studies have been subsequently performed in 8 hypercholesterolemic (type IIa) female subjects. In these subjects a slight but significant reduction in total cholesterol after the treatment with n-3 fatty acids is observed; a reduction of about 30% of triglycerides is also observed; a quite marked reduction of VLDL and a more modest reduction of LDL is also seen (Tab. II). When one compares baseline and post-treatment values in these patients with values of normolipidemic subjects,

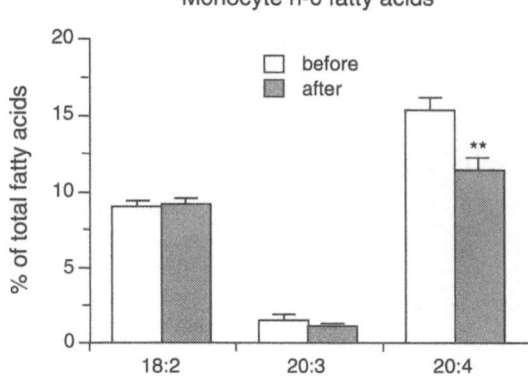

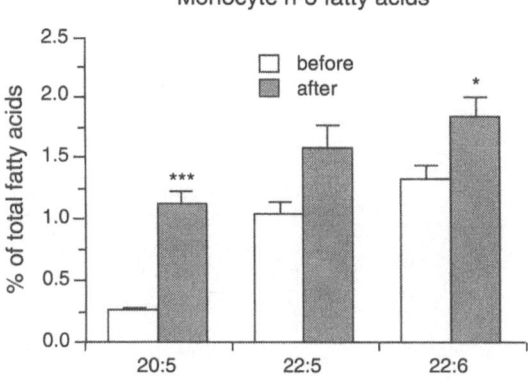

Fig. 3. Levels of n-6 (upper panel) and n-3 (lower panel) fatty acids as percent of total fatty acids in monocyte phospholipids of normolipidemic subjects, before and after treatment. There were significant differences from corresponding values before treatment, at the following levels: * $p<0.05$; ** $p<0.02$; *** $p<0.001$

Table I. Fatty acid ratios (EPA/AA, EPA/DHA) in capsules and in plasma and cells before and after treatment with n-3 fatty acids in male normolipidemics.

		Capsules	Plasma	Platelets	PMN	Monocytes
EPA/AA	- { before		0.076	0.015	0.040	0.017
	after		0.666	0.095	0.160	0.101
EPA/DHA	{ before	1.92	0.52	0.39	0.89	0.19
	after		1.89	1.67	0.98	0.62

Table II. Plasma lipids and lipoproteins in Type IIa hypercholesterolemic females before and after a 6-week treatment with n-3 fatty acids.

	Time 0	6 weeks
Plasma lipid		
Cholesterol	284.5± 8.9	268.0± 9.1**
Triglycerides	132.2±13.8	103.8+13.3**
Lipoprotein lipid		
HDL - Cholesterol	51.9±2.7	53.5± 2.7
- Free cholesterol	10.1±0.9	10.6± 1.0
- Triglycerides	15.6±1.0	13.1± 1.1
- Phospholipids	95.6±4.0	94.7± 2.4
VLDL - Cholesterol	19.7± 2.1	14.7± 2.1**
- Free cholesterol	9.7± 1.2	6.8± 0.9*
- Triglycerides	76.9±11.9	51.5±11.6**
- Phospholipids	27.2± 3.7	24.7± 3.7
LDL - Cholesterol	211.3±8.1	199.9± 8.0*
- Free cholesterol	42.7±3.6	38.0± 3.1
- Triglycerides	45.9±3.6	41.2± 8.7
- Phospholipids	130.4±5.0	129.6± 4.9

Values, expressed as mg/dl, are the average ± SEM
Significance of differences from Time 0: * $p<0.05$, ** $p<0.01$

Table III. Levels of n-6 and n-3 fatty acids in plasma of male volunteers before and after 6-week treatment with n-3 fatty acids.

Fatty Acids	Time 0	6 weeks
	nmoles / ml	
18:2	3234 ± 157	2428 ± 173
20:4	481 ± 36	365 ± 19*
20:5	33 ± 5	221 ± 21**
22:6	66 ± 7	109 ± 7*

Values are the average ± SEM. Values with the asterisk are significantly different from values at Time 0 at the following levels: * $p<0.05$; ** $p<0.01$.

Table IV. Levels of n-6 and n-3 fatty acids in plasma of female hypercholesterolemic subjects before and after 6-week treatment with n-3 fatty acids.

Fatty Acids	Time 0	6 weeks
	nmoles/ml	
18:2	4242±140	3955± 201
20:4	700± 30	618± 31
20:5	95± 10	801± 26**
22:6	136± 14	351± 34*

Values are the average ± SEM. Values with the asterisk are significantly different from values at Time 0 at the following levels: * p< 0.01; ** p<0.001

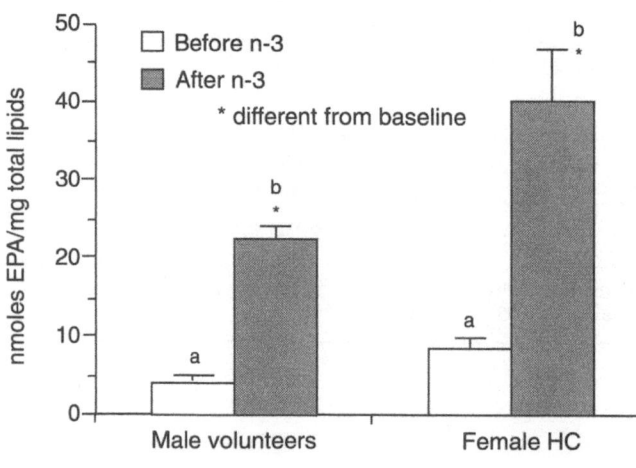

Fig. 4. A comparison of the EPA incorporation into platelet phospholipids of male volunteers (left columns) and hypercholesterolemic females (right columns) after dietary supplementation with equal amounts of n-3 fatty acids (EPA 2.8 g, DHA 1.7 g daily) as ethyl esters for 6 weeks. Values with the same letter are different from each other.

Table V. EPA/AA ratios in plasma and cells of male volunteers (M Vol) and female hypercholesterolemic (FHC) subjects, before (T_0) and after 6-week (T_{6w}) treatment with n-3 fatty acids.

		Plasma		Platelets		PMN		Monocytes	
		T_0	T_{6w}	T_0	T_{6w}	T_0	T_{6w}	T_0	T_{6w}
M.	Vol	0.076	0.666	0.015	0.095	0.040	0.160	0.017	0.101
F.	HC	0.116	1.006	0.025	0.150	0.052	0.275	0.057	0.173

T_0: Time 0; T_{6w}: Time 6 weeks. M=Male; F=Female

it can be clearly seen that plasma levels of EPA and DHA in hypercholesterolemic subjects are much higher than in healthy subjects (Tab. III, IV), and that the incorporation into cell membranes is more evident (Fig. 4 and Tab. V). The reasons for this difference are not clear at the moment. However the increase in EPA incorporation obtained in this study is superimposable on that obtained by other authors[4-5] who have supplemented n-3 fatty acids with triglyceride formulations.

In conclusion, the supplementation of n-3 fatty acids with ethyl ester preparations, although possibly leading to less efficient hydrolysis of the compounds and slower absorption, is suitable to determine an increased incorporation of these fatty acids into cell membranes. A different accumulation pattern is seen in normo- and hypercholesterolemic subjects.

References

1. Bottino N.R., Vandenberg, G.S., Reiser, R.: Resistance of certain long-chain polyunsaturated fatty acids of marine oils to pancreatic lipase. Lipids 1967; 2, 489-493
2. Heimermann W.H., Holman, R.T., Gordon, D.T., Kowalyshyn, D.E., Jensen, R.G.: Effect of double bond positions in octadecanoates upon hydrolysis by pancreatic lipase. Lipids 1973; 8, 45-47
3. Lawson L.D., Hughes B.G.: Human absorption of fish oil fatty acids as triglycerides, free acids, or ethyl esters. Biochem. Biophys. Res. Commun. 1988; 152, 328-335
4. Zucker M.L., Bilyen D.S., Helmkampf G.M., Harris W.S., Dujovne C.A.: Effects of dietary fish oil on platelet function and plasma lipids in hypercholesterolemic and normal subjects. Atherosclerosis 1988; 73, 13-22
5. Harris W.S., Zucker M.L., Dujovne C.A.: Omega-3 fatty acids in hypertriglyceridemic patients: triglycerides vs methyl esters. Am.J.Clin.Nutr. 1988; 48, 992-997
6. Dart A.M., Riemersma R.A., Oliver M.F.: Effects of Maxepa on serum lipids in hypercholesterolemic subjects. Atherosclerosis 1989; 80,119-124

n-3 Fatty Acids and the Vessel Wall

7. n-3 Fatty Acids and Platelet-Vessel Wall Interactions

R. De Caterina
CNR Institute of Clinical Physiology, Pisa, Italy

The protective effects of n-3 fatty acids in vascular atherosclerotic diseases, as shown in a number of epidemiological and experimental studies, have led to the proposition that these compounds may interfere with platelet-vessel wall interactions, a process which is pivotal in the development of thrombosis and, possibly, of atherosclerosis. That n-3 fatty acids interfere with platelet-vessel wall interactions is simply demonstrated by the fact, now established beyond any reasonable doubt, that they are able to prolong the bleeding time. Bleeding time is a "global" test exploring platelet reactions to a standardized interruption of vascular integrity; actually it appears to be the only test practically available to explore these interactions in vivo, in humans, in an integrated way; it suffers however from methodological problems (some variability in technique) and from theoretical flaws: its relationship with actual bleeding in other parts of the body is not proven; its value - on the other hand - as a thrombotic predictor is also unproven; finally, because of its "globality", it does not provide insights into the mechanism(s) involved in its alterations. Therefore a "dissection" of the effects of n-3 fatty acids on platelet-vessel wall interactions requires the analysis of:

1. studies on isolated platelets;
2. studies on the isolated vessel wall;
3. studies of interaction products.

Each of these separate approaches provides a partial insight into the problem, but the information which can be obtained by each of these approaches will be eventually useful to compose a final pattern of mechanistic interpretation. We will distinguish, for the sake of simplicity and according to the historical process on which the mechanism of action of n-3 fatty acids has been traditionally interpreted, two broad groups of possible interference of n-3 fatty acids with platelet-vessel wall interactions, namely eicosanoid-dependent and eicosanoid-independent ("other") mechanisms.

Studies on Isolated Platelets

According to the initial hypothesis of interpretation of the mechanism of action of n-3 fatty acids against thrombosis, as proposed by Dyerberg et al.,[1] their effects on platelet-vessel wall interactions derive from the simple substitution of substrates for the cyclooxygenase and lipooxygenase enzymes. The substitution of eicosapentaenoic acid (EPA) for arachidonic acid (AA) changes the pattern of metabolites of cyclooxygenase, the enzyme normally catalyzing the transformation of AA into prostaglandin cyclic endoperoxides. The metabolism of these endoperoxides is normally oriented towards the formation of platelet thromboxane (TX) A_2, proaggregatory and vasoconstrictive, in platelets, and of prostaglandin (PG) I_2 (prostacyclin), antiaggregatory and vasodilatory, in the vessel wall. When EPA substitutes AA in membrane phospholipids the formation of TXA_3 and of PGI_3 occurs.[2,3] While the latter retains most of the biological properties of PGI_2, TXA_2 is virtually inactive. Therefore the "balance" normally existing between platelet and vessel wall eicosanoids is shifted towards the inhibition of platelet function and vasodilation.

Experimental data, however, now indicate that this hypothesis does not account for the actions of n-3 fatty acids on platelets. Indeed, while platelet production of TXB_2 is reduced under treatment with n-3 fatty acids (Fig. 1), the amount of reduction is usually lower than necessary for an appreciable reduction of platelet function, due to the demonstrated non-linear relationship between reduction of thromboxane production and reduction of aggregation. It has indeed been calculated[4] that more than 90% inhibition of TX is necessary to obtain some inhibition of platelet aggregation.

With n-3 fatty acids, on the other hand, and at variance with aspirin, inhibition of platelet aggregation to weak agonists (such as ADP and adrenaline) can be seen for inhibition of serum TXB_2 less than 50%.[5] Also, the hypothesis of substrate substitution would imply that the amount of $TXA_2 + TXA_3$ does not change. Data from many reported studies show that this simply does not occur. In a recently published study in dogs fed 0.8 g/kg total n-3 per day (an amount corresponding to more than 50 g/day in humans!) total immunoreactive serum TXB ($TXB_2 + TXB_3$) decreased from 693 ± 80 ng/ml to 99 ± 18 ng/ml, about an 86% reduction.[6] Even taking into account TX urinary metabolite excretion, a statistically significant reduction of the total excretion of $TXA_2 + TXA_3$ metabolites is evident.

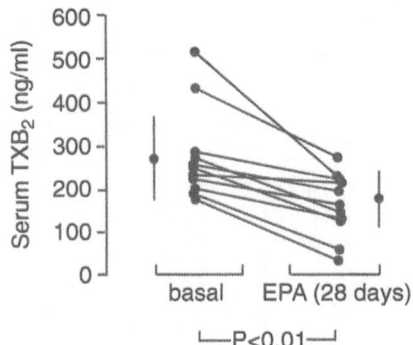

Fig. 1. Serum thromboxane B$_2$ before and after treatment with fish oil (3 g EPA + 1.8 g DHA/day for 28 days) in 15 patients with coronary artery disease. Individual results and mean ± SEM are reported. TXB$_2$ has been measured by radioimmunoassay, with an antibody extensively cross-reacting with TXB$_3$. A clear reduction in serum thromboxane is evident (reprinted from *Circulation*,[5] with permission).

Conclusions can be drawn from such evidence that:

1. the decrease in total immunoreactive serum TXB (an index of the maximum platelet capacity to produce thromboxane) cannot be explained by the hypothesis of substrate substitution;
2. the decrease of TXB$_2$ production by platelets is not able to account for the reduced platelet aggregability ex vivo to a variety of stimuli;
3. the formation of inactive TXB$_3$ does indeed occur, but is only one aspect of eicosanoid modification induced by n-3 fatty acids.

Studies on the Isolated Vessel Wall

Attempts at validating the Dyerberg's hypothesis at the vessel wall level were precluded by the difficulty of measuring the direct production of prostacyclins in humans under fish oil treatment. This was recently made possible in a study in which we were able to measure the production of prostacyclin (by radioimmunoassay of its stable *in vitro* metabolite 6-keto-PGF$_{1\alpha}$) from human vascular fragments *ex vivo* obtained from 14 patients undergoing bypass surgery after a 4-week treatment with fish oil. These were compared with fragments obtained from 15 control patients matched for a number of demographic and clinical variables. Vascular fragments consisted of saphenous veins, aortas and atrial appendages. Saphenous vein fragments were studied also in special incubation chambers to assess the selective endothelial contribution to luminal production of prostacyclin. In all conditions production of prostacyclin from vascular fragments after fish oil treatment was higher than in control conditions (Fig. 2).[5] It should be pointed out that such a measurement, obtained both in unstimulated conditions (mechanical stimulation only) and after exposure to arachidonic acid, is more a "capacity" index than an index of actual production rate, and therefore yields information

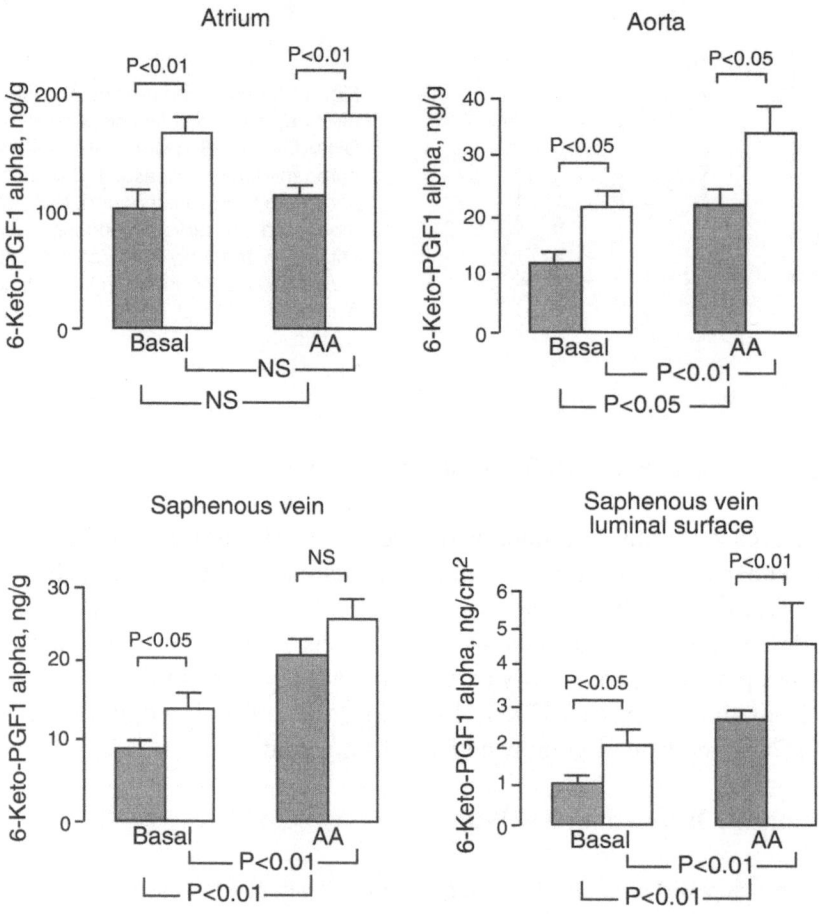

Fig. 2. Production of prostacyclin (6-keto-PGF$_{1a}$, ng/g wet weight of tissue or ng/cm^2 of exposed area) in basal conditions (mechanical stimulation only) and after incubation with arachidonic acid, in control subjects (stippled columns) and subjects treated with fish oil (3 g EPA + 1.8 g DHA/day for 28 days)(white columns). Results are expressed as mean ± SEM. A clear increase in prostacyclin production is evident in all conditions from patients after fish oil treatment (reprinted from *Circulation*,[5] with permission).

equivalent to what is obtainable in platelets from serum thromboxane measurements. On the other hand, measurements of the actual production rate of the vessel wall in vivo, independently of platelet contribution, does not appear to be feasible methodologically in humans. Our measurements, mostly measuring PGI$_2$ and only to a minor extent PGI$_3$, directly contradict the hypothesis of substrate substitution.

In vivo Measurement of Interaction Products

The actual production rate of prostacyclins in vivo, measured by the evaluation of the urinary excretion of prostacyclin metabolites, can be regarded as a true measure of interaction products, since it has been shown that it increases concomitantly with situations of extensive platelet activation, such as severe atherosclerotic vascular disease,[7] probably as a reflection of platelet contribution of substrates for vascular prostacyclin production. In conditions where extensive vascular disease is not present, there is no evidence that metabolites of PGI_2 are decreased after fish oil treatment, while a clear increase of PGI_3 metabolites is always evident.[3,8] Calculations made adding up $PGI_2 + PGI_3$ metabolites from such studies generally indicate at least a trend towards the increase of prostacyclins. On the other hand, this does not appear to occur in situations in which extensive vascular disease is present; in such cases baseline prostacyclin excretion is elevated and the effect of fish oil is generally towards a reduction, which can be explained by a prevailing effect of fish oil on platelet function in these situations of extensive platelet activation, thus reducing platelet contribution to vascular production of prostacyclin. Taken as a whole, again these studies do not appear to support the hypothesis of simple substrate substitution as an explanation for the effects of n-3 fatty acids on platelet-vessel wall interactions.

Probably a rearrangement of cellular pools of arachidonic acid and/or effects on specific enzymes in the eicosanoid pathways occur under treatment with these compounds.

Relevant to the original question posed, however, it would appear that the entire issue of eicosanoid modifications as an explanation for the effects of n-3 fatty acids on platelet-vessel wall interactions has been overemphasized recently. It is interesting to note that a protective effect of fish oils against restenosis after percutaneous transluminal coronary angioplasty (PTCA) has been described at least in some of the studies performed to address this issue.[9-12] PTCA is a condition in which vessel wall intimal tearing and damage by the balloon used to dilate an atherosclerotic stenosis creates extensive enhancement of platelet-vessel wall interactions, which are thought to contribute to the subsequent development of restenosis. If such effect really occurs, it would appear in conditions in which the entire cyclooxygenase arm of the eicosanoid system is almost completely wiped out from the concomitant treatment with aspirin.

Other effects of n-3 fatty acids on platelet-vessel wall interactions not mediated by the eicosanoids would appear therefore to be more important in explaining experimental data. Many such effects have been described, such as the increased vascular formation of nitric oxide,[13] potentially able to affect both platelet function and vasodilation, or other thromboxane-independent inhibition of platelet function; effects on the anticoagulant properties of the vessel wall, such as the decreased expression of tissue factor,[14] able to reduce the potential for thrombin generation in the proximity of the vessel wall surface, could also contribute. Many such effects still require wider confirmation and further studies to better define their pathophysiological relevance.

References

1. Dyerberg J., Bang H.O., Stofferson E., Moncada S., Vane J.R.: Eicosapentaenoic acid and prevention of thrombosis and atherosclerosis. Lancet 1978; 1: 117-119
2. Fischer S., Weber P.C.: Thromboxane A_3 (TXA$_3$) is formed in human platelets after dietary eicosapentaenoic acid (C20:5 ω-3). Biochem Biophys Res Commun 1983; 116: 1091 -1099
3. von Schacky C., Fischer S., Weber P.C.: Long-term effects of dietary marine ω-3 fatty acids upon plasma and cellular lipids, platelet function, and eicosanoid formation in humans. J. Clin. Invest. 1985; 76: 1626-1631
4. Lands W.E.M., Culp B.R., Hirai A., Gorman R.: Relationship of thromboxane generation to the aggregation of platelets from humans: effects of eicosapentaenoic acid. Prostaglandins 1985; 30:819-825
5. De Caterina R., Giannessi D., Mazzone A., Bernini W., Lazzerini G., Maffei S., Cerri M., Salvatore L., Weksler B.: Vascular prostacyclin is increased in patients ingesting ω-3 polyunsaturated fatty acids before coronary artery bypass surgery. Circulation 1990; 82: 428-438
6. Braden G.A., Knapp H.R., Fitzgerald D.J., FitzGerald G.A.: Dietary fish oil accelerates the response to coronary thrombolysis with tissue-type plasminogen activator. Evidence for a modest platelet inhibitory effect in vivo. Circulation 1990; 82: 178-187
7. FitzGerald G.A., Smith B., Pedersen A.K., Brash A.R.: Increased prostacyclin biosynthesis in patients with severe atherosclerosis and platelet activation. N. Engl. J. Med. 1984; 310: 1065-1068
8. Knapp H.R., Reilly I.A.G., Alessandrini P., FitzGerald G.A.: In vivo indexes of platelet and vascular function during fish-oil administration in patients with atherosclerosis. N. Engl. J. Med. 1986; 314: 937-942
9. Slack J.D., Pinkerton C.A., Van Tassel J., Orr C.M., Scott M., Allen B., Nasser W.K.: Can oral fish oil supplement minimize re-stenosis after percutaneous transluminal coronary angioplasty? J. Am. Coll. Cardiol. 1987; 9: 64A
10. Dehmer G.J., Popma J.J., van den Berg E.K., Eichhorn E.J., Prewitt J.B., Campbell W.B., Jennings L., Willerson J.T., Schmitz J.M.: Reduction in the rate of early restenosis after coronary angioplasty by a diet supplemented with n-3 fatty acids. N. Engl. J. Med. 1988; 319: 733-740
11. Milner M.R., Gallino R.A., Leffingwell A., Descalzi Pichard A., Brooks-Robinson S., Rosenberg J., Little T., Lindsay J.: Usefulness of fish oil supplements in preventing clinical evidence of restenosis after percutaneous transluminal coronary angioplasty. Am. J. Cardiol. 1989; 64:294-299
12. Roy L., Bairati I., Meyer F., Genest M.B.: Double-blind randomized controlled trial of fish oil supplements in the prevention of restenoses after coronary angioplasty. Circulation 1991; 11-365 (abstract 14)
13. Shimokawa H., Vanhoutte P.M.: Dietary cod-liver oil improves endothelium dependent responses in hypercholesterolemic and atherosclerotic porcine coronary arteries. Circulation 1988; 78:1421-1430
14. Hansen J.B., Olsen J.O., Wilsgard L., Østerud B.: Effect of dietary supplementation with cod liver oil on monocyte thromboplastin synthesis, coagulation and fibrinolysis. J. Int. Med. 1989; 225-Suppl 1: 133-139

8. Platelets, Leukocytes and Atherosclerosis: Possible Links between n-3 Fatty Acids and Protection from Atherosclerosis

B.B. WEKSLER

Division of Hematology-Oncology, Department of Medicine, Cornell University Medical College, New York, USA

Involvement of Activated Blood Cells in Atherosclerosis

The development of an atheromatous plaque in an artery is a complex process requiring interactions of the vascular wall not only with plasma factors such as lipoproteins but also with multiple cellular elements, the most relevant being platelets and leukocytes.[1] The endothelial lining of an artery normally displays multiple antithrombotic mechanisms that promote blood flow and inhibit clot formation (Tab. I). In contrast, loss of, or damage to endothelium promotes local thrombus formation, leukocyte accumulation, and release of mitogenic factors into the arterial wall. More subtle injury to endothelium (see below) can also promote thrombosis.[2] Endothelial damage and a proliferative response to this injury are frequently involved in the initial stages of atherosclerotic plaque formation, associated with changes in normal antithrombotic properties of the vascular endothelium to favor a "prothrombotic" state. Thus, atherosclerotic plaque formation is promoted by local activation of hemostatic and inflammatory responses at the blood vessel wall.

Roles of Endothelial Injury

Numerous stimuli, including high plasma lipid levels, turbulent flow, injury, infection, or exposure to endotoxin or hypoxia, can induce prothrombotic changes in endothelium.[2] A wide variety of altered vascular functions ensue (Tab. II). The endothelium acquires a capacity to promote local blood coagulation, by expressing tissue factor and by binding and activating coagulation factors IX and X, favoring

Table I. Comparison between anti-thrombotic and prothrombotic functions of normal vascular endothelium. Upregulation of procoagulant functions is commonly associated with injury, infection or inflammation, which also may govern decreases in antithrombotic properties.

Anti-Thrombotic	Procoagulant
PGI$_2$	VWF
Nitric oxide	Binding/activation of coagulation factors
Heparan SO$_4$	Tissue factor
AT III	Cytokines
ADPase	Cell adhesion molecules
tPA	PAF
Fibrinolytic assembly	PDGF
Thrombomodulin	PAI
LACI	

PGI$_2$=prostacyclin; AT III=antithrombin III; tPA=tissue plasminogen activator; LACI=lipid activated coagulation inhibitor; VWF=von Willebrand's factor; PAF=platelet aggregating factor; PDGF=platelet derived growth factor; PAI=plasminogen activator inhibitor

Table II. Atherogenic mechanisms that involve interaction of the blood vessel wall with circulating blood cells and plasma factors.

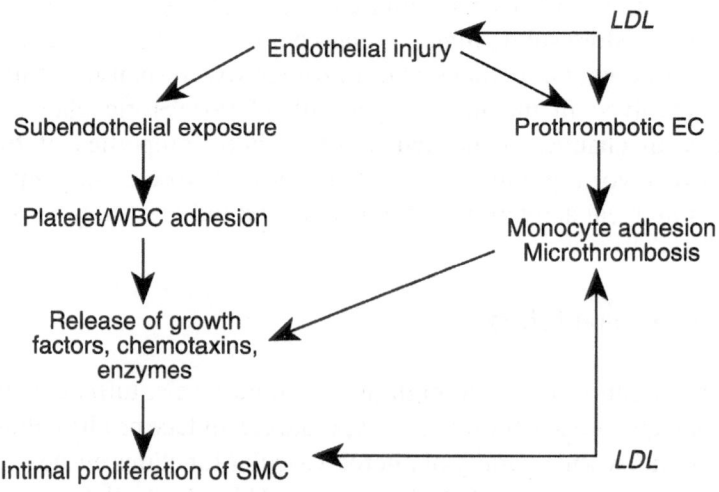

LDL= low density lipoprotein; EC= endothelial cell; SMC= smooth muscle cell; WBC=leukocytes.

deposition of thrombin; von Willebrand's factor is also released. Increased release of plasminogen activator inhibitor (PAI-1) is observed, while thrombomodulin expression and the release of plasminogen activators decrease, thus diminishing effective fibrinolysis.

Involvement of Circulating Blood Cells

Circulating leukocytes are also involved in this process.[3] Activated endothelium expresses membrane glycoproteins such as ICAM-1 and ELAM-1 that are adhesion receptors for ligands present on the membrane of activated leukocytes. Moreover, activated endothelium produces membrane-bound platelet activating factor (PAF) which aggregates leukocytes, and secretes the peptide endothelin, a potent vasoconstrictor and mitogen for smooth muscle cells.

The endothelium produces cytokines, releases platelet derived growth factor (PDGF) a strong chemotaxin for leukocytes and a mitogen for vascular smooth muscle cells, and produces oxygen-derived free radicals and leukotriene C_4. These endothelial changes all favor leukocyte adherence to the arterial wall, altered vascular permeability and leukocyte migration, and the release from leukocytes and platelets of cytokines, growth factors, proteolytic enzymes, free oxygen radicals and eicosanoids. In the presence of hyperlipidemia, the release of cytokines by the endothelium is further enhanced.

The prothrombotic changes in endothelial function that permit localized thrombin generation on the vascular surface as detailed above favor platelet deposition even in the absence of endothelial denudation of the vessel.

In turn, thrombosis on the altered or injured arterial surface also contributes to atherosclerotic plaque formation.

Thrombin itself is mitogenic. Aggregating platelets release growth factors (such as PDGF, EGF, TGFbeta, FGF) that stimulate smooth muscle cell migration and proliferation and enhance matrix protein synthesis. There may also be transfer of platelet-derived cholesterol to smooth muscle cells or macrophages, enhancing foam cell formation.

In the absence of overt physical injury to the endothelium, monocytes (rather than platelets) appear to initiate early atherosclerotic changes. Smooth muscle cells can release chemotactic factors for monocytes.

Monocytes adhere to then migrate across the endothelium to lodge in the subendothelial space, where, if activated, they secrete proteases that release mitogenic factors from the extracellular matrix.[4]

These mitogens induce underlying medial arterial smooth muscle cells to proliferate.

Moreover, monocyte activation is enhanced by hyperlipidemia and by activated platelets.

The *in vivo* relevance of these interactions between blood leukocytes and platelets and the vessel wall is supported by observations made in certain patients with crescendo angina pectoris, a clinical situation that responds particularly well to antiplatelet therapy with aspirin.

Some patients with this syndrome exhibit an inflammatory response in the pericoronary artery tissue located in the territory of the ischemic coronary artery, with an accumulation of PMN and mononuclear cells in the vasa vasorum and perineurally in the coronary adventitia. Production of inflammatory mediators such as leukotriene C_4, thromboxane A_2 and prostacyclin are significantly increased in such areas.[5]

Effects of n-3 Polyunsaturated Fatty Acids

Administration of n-3 fatty acids appears to slow down or to inhibit the formation of experimental atherosclerotic lesions, possibly through their anti-inflammatory effects on components of the lesions.[6] Polyunsaturated fatty acids of the n-3 family alter platelet and leukocyte function in several different ways and also affect vessel wall metabolism (Tab.III).

To understand the mechanisms involved, it is important first to review how the main factors involved in atherogenesis interact in biochemical pathways. These depend upon the type of vascular disturbance incurred.

Table III. Documented modulatory effects of fish oil (and n-3 polyunsaturated fatty acids) on blood components and the vascular endothelium.

Reported positive effects of fish oil or n-3 PUFA

On platelets:	↓ adhesion aggregation TXA_2 synthesis	**On lipids:** ↓	triglycerides
On leukocytes:	↓ chemotaxis LTB_4 inflammation cytokines	**On plasma proteins:** ↓ Fibrinogen PAI ↑ AT III tPA	
On endothelium:	↓ growth factor release cytokines ↑ EDRF (NO) PGI_2 and PGI_3		

In the presence of overt endothelial injury (for example, after angioplasty), platelet activation on the injured surface is a key early event that releases growth factors and chemotaxins and generates thrombin. In this process, close interaction between platelets and neutrophils (or monocytes) occurs.

Platelets produce chemotactic factors for neutrophils and enhance their adherence and aggregation. Platelets or their released products, such as serotonin, augment PMN-induced endothelial injury. PMN elastase activity is enhanced by released platelet factor 4.

Moreover, platelets produce, by interacting with PMN, new eicosanoids that could not be formed by a single isolated cell type.[7] These changes favor migration into the intima and proliferation of vascular smooth muscle cells from the media. Later, monocytes infiltrate the area of the plaque and contribute to its continued development (see above).

In contrast, in the absence of mechanical endothelial injury (for example, in hypercholesterolemia), changes in the endothelial surface properties induce, at a very early stage, the attachment of monocytes which penetrate the endothelium and can initiate proliferative responses by inducing release of growth factors in the absence of platelet contributions.

Antiplatelet Effects of n-3 Fatty Acids

n-3 fatty acids affect both circulating cells in the blood and cells in the vessel wall by mechanisms that mitigate atherogenesis. These compounds, administered as dietary supplements of several grams per day, decrease platelet aggregation and release of thromboxane A_2 and block the TXA_2 receptor on platelets.[8]

They also favor reduction of platelet adhesion to fibrinogen and collagen, an effect that is independent from the eicosanoid system and which appears rather to be mediated by synthesis of nitric oxide, the endothelium-derived relaxing factor.[9] The effect on platelets has been confirmed by measuring prolongation of platelet survival in patients with atherosclerosis, who untreated often show some shortening of platelet survival thought due to repeated platelet activation.[10]

Modulation of Leukocyte Function by n-3 Fatty Acids

n-3 fatty acids reduce neutrophil chemotaxis in healthy subjects and in patients with ischemic heart disease in a reversible manner.[11,12]

In addition, neutrophil adherence to endothelial cells, like platelet adherence to adhesive proteins on other platelets, is diminished during treatment with n-3 fatty acids over a period of 1-3 weeks.[13]

Important interactions between platelets and monocytes may also be regulated by n-3 fatty acids. Platelets bind to monocytes, produce chemotactic factors for monocytes, augment monocyte adherence, stimulate tissue factor production, and alter the monocyte pattern of eicosanoid production. Platelets may also enhance macrophage cholesterol content, favoring the transformation of the monocyte-derived macrophages into foam cells. n-3 fatty acids significantly reduce cytokine production by macrophages, inhibit a variety of growth factors, and can reduce the synthesis by endothelial cells of PDGF.[14-16]

n-3 Fatty Acids and Control of Intimal Hyperplasia

In dog models of vascular autografts, n-3 fatty acids decrease mitogen release by monocytes, reduce serum mitogenic activity after grafting, and increase the production of nitric oxide from endothelial cells.[17]

Nitric oxide has been shown to inhibit vascular smooth muscle cell proliferation. In similar vascular graft models, the net effect of the multiple mechanisms by which n-3 fatty acids inhibit atherogenesis is a decrease in post-grafting intimal hyperplasia.[18]

Comparison of the effects of n-3 fatty acids and of aspirin or thromboxane synthase inhibitors in these models showed that n-3 fatty acids had the greatest effect in decreasing intimal hyperplasia, aspirin alone had a small effect, and thromboxane inhibition was not effective.

Efficacy of treatment did not correlate with inhibition of thromboxane synthesis, suggesting that eicosanoids may not be important factors in supporting arterial smooth muscle proliferation.

Clearly, the antiatherogenic effect of n-3 fatty acids is multifactorial (Tab. III). Direct blocking or redirecting effects upon eicosanoid metabolites produced by blood cells or by the vessel wall represent only one component of n-3 fatty acids' actions.[8]

Inhibition of platelet function by n-3 fatty acids is partial and cannot fully account for anti-atherogenic effects.[18] Anti-inflammatory effects of n-3 fatty acids upon monocyte/macrophage function, first described in the setting of arthritis, also are contributory, especially where cytokine release is an important pathogenic component.

Moreover, n-3 fatty acids may directly alter the function of the blood vessel wall itself, to enhance formation of antithrombotic prostanoids[19] and of nitric oxide,[20] and to block smooth muscle cell proliferation.[21]

These combined anti-atherosclerotic effects of n-3 fatty acids on circulating leukocytes and platelets and on cells of the blood vessel wall are, furthermore, complemented and influenced by their lipid-lowering actions.[16,11,19,22] Thus, n-3 fatty acids provide inhibitory effects at multiple levels not only to block initiation but also to prevent or slow progression of atherosclerosis.

References

1. Ross R.: The pathogenesis of atherosclerosis. New Engl. J. Med. 1986; 314:488-500
2. Gerlach H., Esposito C., Stern D.: Modulation of endothelial hemostatic properties: an active role in the host response. Ann. Rev. Med. 1990; 41: 15-24
3. Pober J.S., Cotran R.S.: The role of endothelial cells in inflammation. Transplantation 1990; 50: 537-544
4. Falcone D.J., McCaffrey T.A., Vergilio J., Haimovitz-Friedman A.: Plasminogen-dependent release of basic fibroblast growth factor (bFGF) from extracellular matrix by foam cells. Ninth International Symposium on Atherosclerosis, International Atherosclerosis Society. Rosemont. IL., 1991; p. 98
5. Weksler B.B., Lloyd-Jones D., Nguyen T., Wallsh E.: Eicosanoid production correlates with leukocytic infiltrate in coronary adventitial biopsies from patients with unstable angina. Blood 1987: 70: 412A
6. Kinsella J.E., Lokesh B., Stone R.A.: Dietary n-3 polyunsaturated fatty acids and amelioration of cardiovascular disease: possible mechanisms. Am. J. Clin. Nutr. 1990; 52: 1-28
7. Marcus A.J.: Thrombosis and inflammation as multicellular processes: pathophysiologic significance of transcellular metabolism. Blood 1990; 76: 1903-1907
8. Swann P.G., Venton D.L., LeBreton G.C.: Eicosapentaenoic acid and docosahexaenoic acid are antagonists at the thromboxane A2/prostaglandin H_2 receptor in human platelets. FEBS Letters 1989; 243: 244-246
9. Li X., Steiner M.: Fish oil: a potent inhibitor of platelet adhesiveness. Blood 1990; 76:938-945
10. Levine P.H., Fisher M., Schneider P.B., Whitten R.H., Weiner B.H., Ockene I.S., Johnson B.F., Johnson M.H., Doyle E.M., Riendeau P.A., Hoogasian J.J.: Dietary supplementation with omega-3 fatty acids prolongs platelet survival in hyperlipidemic patients with atherosclerosis. Arch Int Med 1989; 149: 1113-1116
11. Schmidt E.B., Pedersen J.O., Varming K., Ernst E., Jersild C., Grunnet N., Dyerberg J.: n-3 fatty acids and leukocyte chemotaxis. Effects in hyperlipidemia and dose-response studies in healthy men. Arteriosclerosis and Thrombosis 1991; 11:429-435
12. Mehta J.L., Lopez L., Lawson D., Wargovich T.J., Williams L.L.: Dietary supplementation with omega-3 polyunsaturated fatty acids in patients with stable coronary heart disease. Am. J. Med. 1988; 84:45-52
13. Lee T.H., Hoover R.L., Williams J.D. et al.: Effect of dietary enrichment with eicosapentaenoic and docosahexaenoic acids on in vitro neutrophil and monocyte leukotriene generation and neutrophil function. N. Engl. J. Med. 1985; 312:1217-1224
14. Endres S., Ghorbani R., Kely V.E., Georgilis K., Lonnemenn G., van der Meer J.W., Cannon J.G., Rogers T.S., Klempner M.S., Weber P.C., Schaefer E.J., Wolff S.M., Dinarello C.A.: The effect of dietary supplementation with n-3 polyunsaturated fatty acids on the synthesis of interleukin-1 and tumor necrosis factor by mononuclear cells. New Engl. J. Med. 1989; 320: 265-271
15. Smith D.L., Willis A.I., Nguyen N., Onner D., Zahedi S., Fuks J.: Eskimo plasma constituents, dihomo-gamma-linolenic acid, eicosapentaenoic acid and docosahexaenoic acid, inhibit the release of atherogenic mitogens. Lipids 1989; 24:70-75
16. Fox P.L., DiCorleto P.E.: Fish oils inhibit endothelial cell production of platelet-derived growth factor-like protein. Science 1988; 241:453-466
17. Sarris G.E., Fann J.I., Sokoloff M.H., Smith D.L., Loveday M., Kosek J., Stephens R.J., Cooper A., May K., Willis A.L., Miller D.C.: Mechanisms responsible for inhibition of vein-graft arteriosclerosis by fish oil. Circulation 1989; 80 (suppl I): 1109-1123
18. Sarris G.E., Mitchell R.S., Billingham M.H., Glasson J., Cahill P.D., Miller D.C. Inhibition of

58

accelerated cardiac allograft arteriosclerosis by fish oil. J Thorac Cardiovasc Surg 1989; 97: 841-855

19. DeCaterina R., Giannessi D., Mazzone A., Bernini W., Lazzerini G., Maffei S., Cerri M., Salvatore L., Weksler B.B.: Vascular prostacyclin is increased in patients ingesting omega-3 polyunsaturated fatty acids before coronary artery bypass graft surgery. Circulation 1990; 82: 428-438

20. Shimokawa H., VanHoutte P.M.: Dietary n-3 fatty acids and endothelium-dependent relaxations in porcine coronary arteries. Amer. J. Physiol. 1989; 256: H968-H973

21. Diskin C.J., Thomas C.E., Zellner C.P., Lock S., Tanja J.: Fish oil to prevent intimal hyperplasia and excess thrombosis. Nephron 1990; 55: 445-447

22. Leaf A., Weber P.C.: Cardiovascular effects of n-3 fatty acids. New Engl. J. Med. 1988; 318: 549-557

9. Cytokines and their Modulation by n-3 Fatty Acids with Regard to Atherogenesis

S. ENDRES
Medizinische Klinik, Klinikum Innenstadt der Universität München, Munich, Federal Republic of Germany

Recent data have shown that, among the possible mediators of the pathophysiological mechanisms responsible for atherogenesis in vivo, cytokines may play a major role.[1] Cytokines are secreted proteins that have been initially identified as products of fibroblasts or leukocytes; they act as intercellular signals regulating the function of different cell types and, particularly, their proliferation and differentiation. Figure 1 summarizes the different families of cytokines that have been identified. Nine different types of interleukins (IL) have been isolated so far, as well as two different tumor necrosis factors (TNF) and a variety of other substances such as colony stimulating factors, interferons, transforming growth factors (TGF) and platelet derived growth factors (PDGF).

IL-1 has a variety of effects on endothelial cells, which are depicted in figure 2.[2] Among them, IL-1 potentiates procoagulant activity, increases the production of Plasminogen Activator Inhibitor (PAI) and endothelin, as well as the formation of eicosanoids. Also, this substance augments the adhesion of polymorphonuclear leukocytes, T- and B-cells to endothelial cells. Finally, IL-1 increases the permeability of endothelial cells, a mechanism that appears to be responsible for diabetic nephropathy. These effects may trigger feedback mechanisms that further potentiate IL-1 action on the different cell types (Fig. 3).[3] Thus IL-1 orchestrates a cascade of cellular and biochemical events that lead to vascular congestion, clot formation and

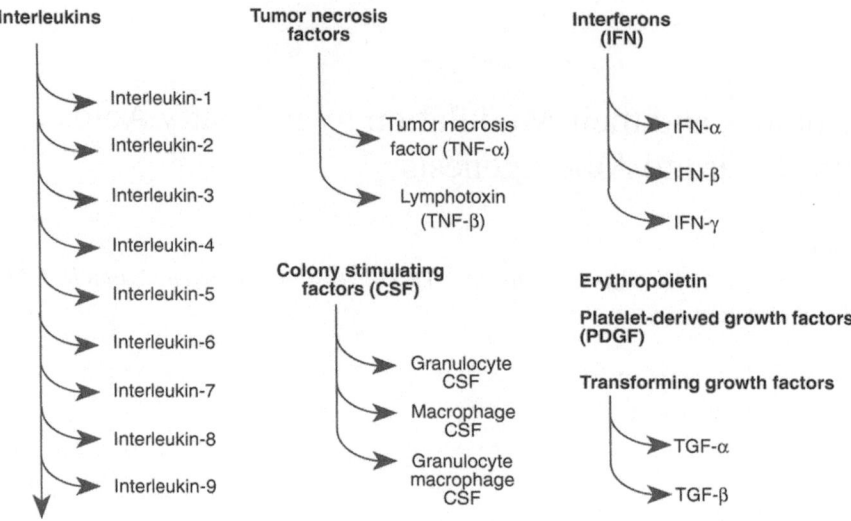

Fig. 1. The cytokine families, in an overview of the nomenclature.

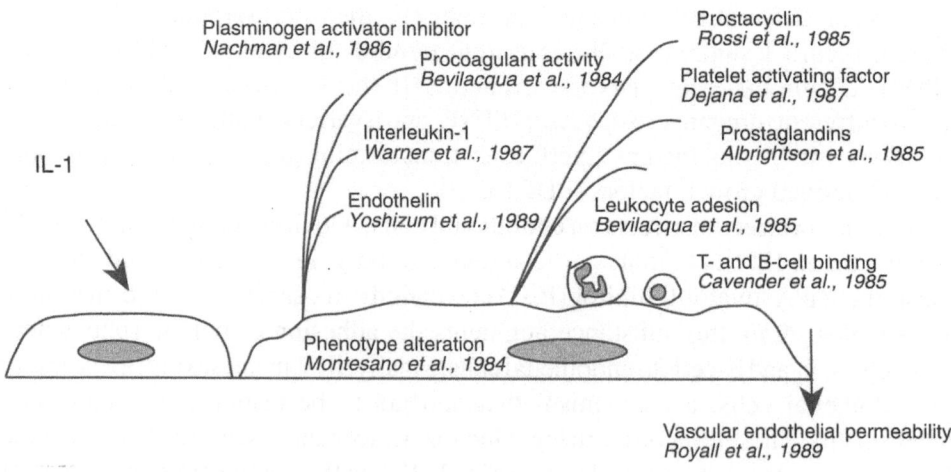

Fig. 2. Effects of interleukin-1 on vascular endothelial cells.[6]

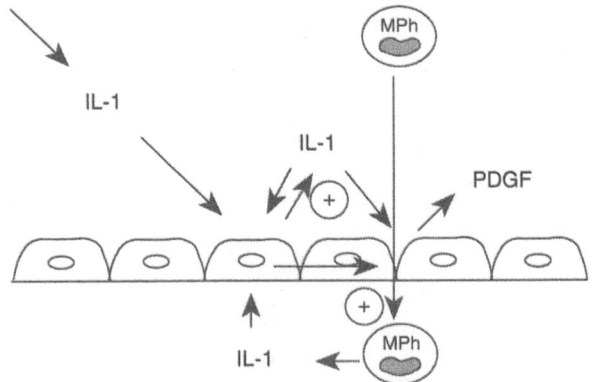

Fig. 3. Possible enhancement mechanisms of interleukin-1 synthesis and action in the vessel wall.

cellular infiltration. All these actions have been demonstrated in preparations in vitro. However, recent evidence indicates that, for example, TNF is present in human atheroma, suggesting that these mediators may indeed play a role in the pathogenesis of atherosclerosis in vivo.[4] Many studies have analyzed the possible mechanisms responsible for the protective effects of n-3 fatty acids against the development of atherosclerosis. The vascular effects of IL-1 and TNF suggest that the production of these pro-inflammatory substances might be a target for the effects of n-3 fatty acids, besides their effects on platelet function, on the eicosanoid system and on plasma lipids. To date the only known pharmacologic agents to reduce cytokine synthesis are corticosteroids and cyclosporine A. We have completed a study to investigate whether dietary supplementation with n-3 fatty acids contained in fish oils affects the synthesis of IL-1 and TNF. Since IL-1 and TNF are principal mediators of inflammation, reduced production of these cytokines may contribute to the amelioration of inflammatory symptoms in patients taking n-3 supplementation.[5] Nine healthy volunteers received 16g of fish oil per day (corresponding to 4.8 g of eicosapentaenoic acid [EPA] plus docosahexaenoic acid [DHA]) for a period of 6 weeks). Production of IL-1 was measured by a radioimmunoassay after the incubation of mononuclear cells (monocytes plus lymphocytes) for 20 h with a suitable stimulus (e.g. 10 ng/ml of lipopolysaccharide). At the end of the incubations the cells were disrupted by freeze-thaw cycles, thus collecting both cell-associated and secreted cytokines. This *ex-vivo* synthesis of cytokines was significantly reduced. The reduction persisted up to 10 weeks after n-3 fatty acid supplementation, with values returning to baseline 20 weeks after ending the supplement (Fig. 4). Data for TNF were very similar. The measurement of the membrane content of n-3 and n-6 fatty acids showed that therapy had altered the arachidonic acid (AA)/EPA ratio, indicating that the substitution of AA by EPA was associated with the reduced synthesis of these pro-inflammatory proteins.

n-3 fatty acids may also reduce the production of other important mediators. For

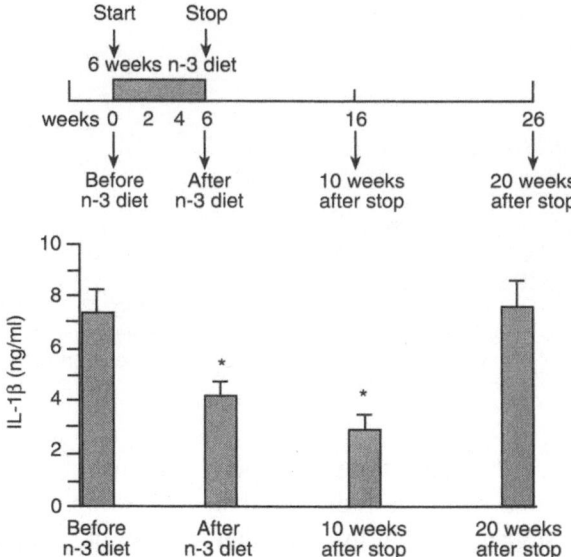

Fig. 4. Influence of n-3 fatty acids on production of IL-1β induced by endotoxin. Mononuclear cells were incubated for 24 hours with 1 ng/ml of endotoxin. IL-1β was determined by RIA. The bars represent the mean values for nine volunteers with error bars as the standard error of the mean. * indicates significant differences from the baseline (before n-3 diet) at p<0.05.

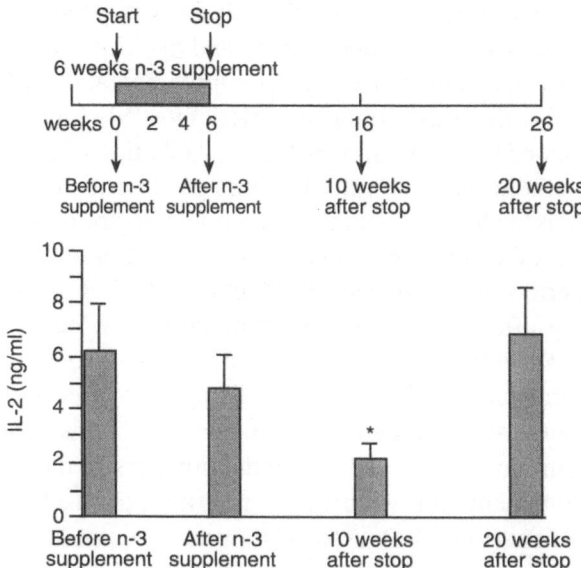

Fig. 5. Influence of n-3 fatty acids on production of IL-2 induced by Phytohemagglutinin. Mononuclear cells were incubated for 24 hours with 3 μg/ml of endotoxin. IL-2 was determined by ELISA. The bars represent the mean values for nine volunteers with error bars as the standard error of the mean. * indicates significant difference from the baseline (before n-3 diet) at p<0.05.

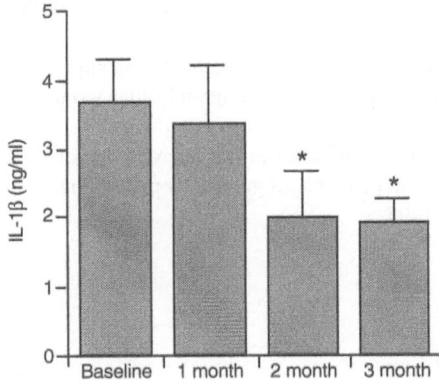

Fig. 6. Effects of a low (2.4 g/d) dosage of n-3 fatty acids for a long period of time (1, 2 and 3 months) on production of IL-1β (by mononuclear cells stimulated with 1 ng/ml of LPS).

example, they were shown to decrease the PMA-induced production of IL-2 (Fig. 5). The above findings were obtained by employing high dosages of n-3 fatty acids for a relatively short period of time. Thus, the effect of a lower dosage of n-3 fatty acids (2.4 g/day) for a longer period of time (3 months) in humans was tested. Results were quite similar; indeed, after 3 months of therapy, a 50% reduction of IL-1 synthesis was observed (Fig. 6).

Mechanisms responsible for the n-3 fatty acid-induced reduction of IL-1 and TNF are still not completely understood. However, a likely mechanism is reduced synthesis of PGE_2: at low concentrations, this eicosanoid has been shown to increase cytokine production through a cyclic AMP-mediated mechanism.[7]

In conclusion, these results demonstrate that n-3 fatty acids may inhibit the production of cytokines. This effect persists up to 10 weeks after ending the treatment. The anti-inflammatory effect of n-3 fatty acids may be mediated in part by decreased cytokine synthesis. Since the vessel wall forms both a cardinal target tissue and a source of cytokines, a suppressive effect on their generation by a n-3 supplemented diet may contribute to its protective effect against atherosclerosis.

References

1. Cotran R.S., Pober J.S.: Effects of cytokines on vascular endothelium: Their role in vascular and immune injury. Kidney Internat. 1989; 35: 969-75
2. Dinarello C.A.: Interleukin-1. Rev. Infect. Dis. 1988; 10:168-89
3. Warner S.J.C., Auger K.R., Libby P.: Human interleukin-1 induces interleukin-1 gene expression in human vascular smooth muscle cells. J. Exp. Med. 1987; 165:1316-21
4. Barath P., Fishbein M.C., Cao J., Berenson J., Helfant R.H., Forrester J.S.: Detection and localisation of tumor necrosis factor in human atheroma. Am. J. Cardiol. 1990; 65:297-302
5. Endres S., Ghorbani R., Kelley V.E., Georgilis K., Lonnemann G., van der Meer J.W.M., Cannon J.G., Rogers T.S., Klempner M.S., Weber P.C., Schaefer E.J., Wolff S.M., Dinarello C.A.: The effect of dietary supplementation with n-3 polyunsaturated fatty acids on the synthesis of

64

interleukin-1 and tumor necrosis factor by mononuclear cells. N. Engl. J. Med. 1989; 320:265-71

6. Meydani S.N., Endres S., Woods M.M. et al.: Oral n-3 fatty acid supplementation suppresses cytokine production and lymphocyte proliferation: comparison in young and older women. J. Nutrition 1991; 121: 547-55

7. Renz H., Gong J.H., Schmidt A., Nain M., Gemsa D.: Release of tumor necrosis factor from macrophages. Enhancement and suppression are dose-dependently regulated by prostaglandin E_2 and cyclic nucleotides. J. Immunol. 1988; 141:2388-93

10. The Effect of n-3 Fatty Acids on Blood Coagulation

G. HORNSTRA

Department of Human Biology, Limburg University, Maastricht, The Netherlands

Introduction

Blood coagulation is likely to play an important role in development and complications of ischaemic heart and vessel disease. This is indicated by the fact that the atherosclerotic plaque contains fibrin,[1] the end product of the coagulation cascade. Moreover, oral anticoagulants appeared to be effective in the secondary prevention of myocardial infarction.[2] Finally, there is strong epidemiological evidence that increased plasma levels of certain coagulation factors are associated with a higher risk of cardiovascular mortality.[3,4]

Activated platelets stimulate blood coagulation;[5] furthermore, thrombin, the central enzyme in coagulation, is an extremely potent activator of blood platelets.[6] Because of these observations, it seems useful to evaluate the influence of dietary n-3 fatty acids on blood coagulation.

The Process of Blood Coagulation

The functional reaction in blood coagulation is the transformation of (soluble) fibrinogen into (insoluble) fibrin. This is accomplished by thrombin, which is formed from an inactive precursor, prothrombin, by the activated form of clotting factor X. Factor Xa can be formed from its inactive precursor factor X by the intrinsic and extrinsic pathways of coagulation, respectively. The intrinsic pathway involves many different coagulation (co)factors and its activity can be quantified by the activated partial thromboplastin time (APTT). Extrinsic clotting involves tissue factor and factor VII and can be evaluated by using the prothrombin time (PT) measurement. The common pathway of blood coagulation (formation of thrombin and fibrin) requires the presence of negatively-charged phospholipids (provided by activated blood platelets) and the factors Va and VIIIa. This common pathway can be measured with the Stypven time and the thrombin time.

Blood coagulation *in vivo* is controlled by a number of natural anticoagulants present in blood plasma and the vessel wall. Two of these substances, antithrombin III and protein C, have been investigated in connection with fish (oil) consumption. These physiological anticoagulants have been shown to be of importance in the "natural defence" against thrombosis, since a deficiency leads to a prothrombotic state.[7,8]

Animal Experiments

Studies with rats showed that the blood plasma of animals fed cod-liver oil for three months was less responsive to the pro-coagulatory activity of a damaged arterial wall than plasma from animals fed sunflowerseed oil-enriched diets.[9] This decreased responsiveness was associated with a prolongation of the prothrombin time (PT) as well as the activated partial thromboplastin time (APTT), which is indicative of a diminished activity of both the extrinsic and intrinsic coagulation systems, respectively.

However, it is unlikely that this is the only explanation for the observed phenomenon, as diets enriched with a more saturated type of fish oil did induce a similar reduction of extrinsic and intrinsic coagulation, but did not or only marginally reduce vessel wall-induced clotting, despite a significantly lower fibrinogen concentration of the plasma. Both types of fish oil caused higher AT-III activities in plasma in comparison to a control group fed a low-fat diet, but the fish oil with the higher saturated fatty acid content was less active than the cod-liver oil in this respect. Both fish oils, however, were less active than sunflowerseed oil with regard to this effect.

These studies demonstrate the existence of physiological effects of dietary fats on blood coagulation. However, rabbits fed the same "saturated" fish oil as used before for the rats, did not show significant differences in extrinsic coagulation (PT), intrinsic blood clotting (APTT) and AT-III activity as compared with animals given either olive-, sunflowerseed-, palm-, or linseed oil in otherwise identical diets for 1.5 years.

Only the plasma fibrinogen content of the fish oil group was somewhat decreased (unpublished results). This difference in effect of the same type of fish oil in two animal studies may be explained by species-differences between rat and rabbit. Alternatively, it is also possible that effects occurring in a short-term dietary study (rat) disappear after a longer period (rabbit). These considerations are also relevant for the interpretation of the human studies to be discussed below.

Human Epidemiology

Epidemiological data (which reflect long-term dietary habits) suggest only marginal effects of fish oil-enriched diets on blood coagulation. Traditionally-living Eskimos do not differ from a comparable Danish control group as to the coagulability of their blood plasma (PT and APTT), notwithstanding a higher fibrinogen content, a higher AT-III content and activity, and a higher content (but not activity) of protein C.[10-13]

Human Intervention Trials

Overall measurements of coagulability

The epidemiologic observations are in accordance with most human intervention studies. With a few exceptions[14,15] the enrichment of human diets with fish, fish oil or a fish oil concentrate did not have measurable effects on PT[16-20] and APTT.[15-19,21,22]

Coagulation times of citrated blood after recalcification,[23] whole-blood clotting time,[24] and thrombin time[25] were also unaffected.

Plasma fibrinogen

Large-scale epidemiological studies indicate that the plasma fibrinogen content is a powerful risk indicator for ischaemic vascular disease.[3,4]

On the great majority of intervention trials, plasma fibrinogen levels are not significantly affected by dietary fish (oil).[17-21,25-29] In one study, however, an increase was seen in the plasma fibrinogen content.[30] In another study, a daily dose of 14 g of a fish oil concentrate, administered for 6 weeks (ca. 6.5g n-3 fatty acids per day), resulted in a significant reduction of the plasma fibrinogen level.[31]

The effect was maximal after 3 weeks and tended to normalize (but was still significant) after 6 weeks. No significant effect was observed in a control group, receiving olive oil. At a considerably lower dose (2.2 or 1.1 g fish oil per day, given for 20 weeks) plasma fibrinogen content has also been reported to be reduced considerably.[32]

Ten ml fish oil (1.8 g of n-3 fatty acids) per day given to angina pectoris patients for a period of 4 years, resulted in a consistent reduction of the plasma fibrinogen content by about 23% over the 4 year period.[33] Thus, the effect of dietary fish (oil) on the plasma content of fibrinogen is inconsistent and requires further careful studies.

Factor VII and VIIa

Clotting factor VII has been shown to be a powerful risk indicator for ischaemic cardiovascular disease.[3] The effect of dietary fish (oil) on factor VII is, again, inconsistent. In most studies no effects were observed.[18,24,27-30] In one (uncontrolled) study a decrease was seen,[17] whereas in non-insulin-dependent diabetics, the daily consumption of 10 g fish oil for 6 weeks resulted in a significant increase in the plasmatic factor Vll activity as compared to the same amount of olive oil.[34]

Administration of a fish-oil concentrate, containing a very high concentration (67%) of the ethyl ester of timnodonic acid, induced a significant increase of the circulating amount of activated factor VII at the expense of non-activated factor VII.[9] This points to an enhanced consumption of factor VII as a result of *in-vivo* activation.

Other clotting factors

In most studies, dietary fish (oil) was shown to have no effect on the plasma concentrations of coagulation factors II,[17,21,27] V,[24] VIII$_c$,[24,27-30] VIII von Willebrand,[18] VIII-related antigen,[26,27,35] X[27,30,34] and XII.[22] In one study, however, an increase was seen in the (chromogenic) factor X activity.[30]

This latter finding was confirmed for mackerel consumption.[18] In hyperlipidaemic subjects, the daily administration of 6 g n-3 fatty acids for 6 weeks lowered von Willebrand factor activity.[28]

Administration of 900 mg n-3 fatty acids (as MaxEPA) per day for 30 days resulted in one study in a significant reduction of the coagulation factors V, IX, X, XI and XII.[17] Unfortunately, the study was totally uncontrolled and cannot, therefore, be properly interpreted.

Clot-promoting effect of activated blood platelets

The influence of dietary fish oil on the clot-promoting activity of blood platelets (the so-called PF-3 activity) has been investigated only twice. In an acute study, comparing the effect of a single dose of 100 g of cod-liver oil with that of 100 g of milk fat,[36] the recalcification time of citrated platelet-rich plasma increased significantly by the milk fat, but remained unchanged by the cod-liver oil. This indicates that cod-liver oil, in contrast to milk fat, does not increase PF-3 activity. The PF-3 activity of "washed" thrombocytes was also not influenced by the cod-liver oil.

This activity was significantly decreased, however, by 100 g of milk fat. Since, under these circumstances, the coagulability of citrated platelet-rich plasma increased, the authors postulated that the pro-coagulant activity of platelets after a large intake of milk fat is based on the release of PF-3 from platelets into plasma. However, further analysis of the platelet-poor plasma is required before this explanation can be accepted.

In another study, the daily administration of 30 ml cod-liver oil for 6 weeks to hypercholesterolaemic patients did not affect platelet procoagulant activity, as measured by a PF-3 test in the presence as well as in the absence of factor V.[24]

Clot-promoting effects of macrophages and monocytes

Upon activation, monocytes and macrophages express a thromboplastin-like activity at their surface that may present a nidus for local fibrin formation. Earlier studies demonstrated that sperm whale oil, when fed to rats, reduced this clot-promoting activity of spleen macrophages *in vitro*.[37]

This effect was not observed after feeding sunflowerseed oil, rich in linoleic acid. In contrast, mackerel oil feeding resulted in an enhanced clot-promoting activity of peritoneal macrophages *in vitro* as compared to sunflowerseed oil and a saturated dietary fat (hydrogenated coconut oil).

A viral infection increased the clot-promoting effect of intraperitoneal macrophages. This effect was less pronounced for the macrophages from the fish oil fed animals, as a result of which the differences between the dietary groups disappeared (unpublished results).

The group of Østerud measured the clot-promoting effect of monocytes upon activation with LPS, either or not in the presence or absence of liposomes. In males and females, dietary cod liver oil caused a significant reduction of this procoagulant effect.[38]

Antithrombin III and Protein C

Experimental results with regard to AT-III activity are equivocal: a decrease of AT-III activity has been described following the administration of 20 ml cod-liver oil per day for 6 weeks.[27] In another study, however, the AT-III content (immunological activity) increased significantly following the administration of the fish oil preparation MaxEPA (10 ml/day for 4 weeks), but this did not result in a significant elevation of AT-III activity.[21] In this study, the AT-III content and activity did increase upon the daily administration of 10 ml of a vegetable oil mixture, rich in linoleic acid.

Administration of the ethyl esters of a cod-liver oil concentrate increased the immunoreactive AT-III significantly but did not change AT-III activity.[13] A comparable preparation, given to normal volunteers in an amount of 0.9 g per day for 2-4 weeks, did not change plasma AT-III content.[20] Comparable results were obtained when insulin dependent diabetics were given n-3 PUFAs for periods up to 6 weeks.[29,30] The daily administration of 1-2 g of a fish oil concentrate for 20 weeks did not alter plasma AT-III activity.[32] In addition, protein C antigen remained the same. In another study, however, the daily administration of 900 mg marine n-3 fatty acids for 30 days resulted in a significant reduction of protein C and AT-III antigen levels.[17] Since the study was uncontrolled and comprised only 9 volunteers, its validity is rather limited.

In Type IIa hyperlipidaemic subjects, the daily administration of 6 g n-3 fatty acids for 6 weeks resulted in a significant increase in protein C, whereas in Type IV patients a significant reduction occurred.[28] In the same study, no effect on AT-III activity was observed.

These studies do not support the suggestion, derived from epidemiological data, that a fish (oil) enriched nutrition will increase the physiological anti-coagulatory process via an increased AT-III activity.[11,13] As Eskimos, who emigrated to Denmark, maintain their elevated AT-III activity,[13] this elevation seems to be determined more by genetic than by environmental (nutritional) factors.

Concluding Remarks

From the studies presented here, it can be concluded that dietary fish (oil) may have some effect on factors involved in blood coagulation. However, the effects seem rather limited and the literature is quite equivocal with respect to most of them. The studies reported so far were aimed mainly at measuring the levels of clotting factors in plasma *in vitro*. The relevance of this approach is questionable, however, since these factors circulate in excessive amounts in the blood as inactive zymogens. More studies are required with respect to circulating activated clotting factors. In addition, new techniques are now becoming available to quantitate low-level ongoing coagulation *in vivo* (by measuring activation peptides and enzyme - inhibitor complexes). The use of these techniques is indispensable to obtain reliable information with respect to the influence of dietary n-3 fatty acids on blood coagulation.

References

1. Woolf, N.: Pathology of Atherosclerosis. *Thrombosis and atherosclerosis*. London, Butterworth Scientific 1982; 217-259
2. Vries W.A., de Tijssen J.P.G., Loeliger E.A., Roos J.: A double-blind trial to assess long-term anticoagulant therapy in elderly patients after myocardial infarction. Lancet 1980; 2: 989-994
3. Wilhelmsen L., Svardsudd K., Korsan-Bengtsen K., Larsson B., Welin L., Tibblin G.: Fibrinogen as a risk factor for stroke and myocardial infarction. New. Engl. J. Med. 1984; 311: 501-505
4. Meade T.W., Brozovic M., Chakrabarti R.R., Hannes A.P., Imeson J.D., Mellows S., Miller G.J., North W.R.S., Stirling Y., Thompson S.G.: Haemostatic function and ischaemic heart disease: principal results of the Northwick Park Heart Study. Lancet 1986; 2: 533-537
5. Bevers E.M., Rosing J., Zwaal R.F.A.: Platelets and coagulation. In: MacIntyre D.E., Gordon J. (Eds.): *Platelets in Biology and Pathology III*. Amsterdam, Elsevier Science Publishers, B.V. Biomedical Division 1987; 127-160
6. Davey M.G., Luscher E.F.: Actions of thrombin and other coagulant and proteolytic enzymes on blood platelets. Nature 1967; 216: 857-858
7. Rosenberg R.D., Rosenberg J.S.: Natural anticoagulant mechanisms. J. Clin. Invest. 1984; 74:1-6
8 Broekmans A.W., Veltkamp J.J., Bertina R.M.: Congenital protein C deficiency and venous thromboembolism. A study in three Dutch families. New. Engl. J. Med. 1983; 309: 340-344
9. Hornstra G.: Dietary fats, prostanoids and arterial thrombosis. *Chapter 7: Effect of fish oil feeding on arterial thrombosis, platelet function and blood coagulation*. The Hague, Martinus Nijhoff Publishers, 1982; 106-137

71

10. Dyerberg J., Bang H.O.: Haemostatic function and platelet polyunsaturated fatty acids in Eskimos. Lancet 1979; 2: 433-435
11. Jorgensen K.A., Nielsen A.H., Dyerberg J.: Hemostatic factors and renin in Greenland Eskimos on a high eicosapentaenoic acid intake. Acta Med. Scand. 1986; 219: 473-479
12 Schmidt E.B., Sorensen P.J., Ernst E., Kristensen S.D., Pedersen J.O., Dyerberg J.: Studies on coagulation and fibrinolysis in Greenland Eskimos. Thromb. Res. 1989; 56: 553-558
13. Stoffersen E., Jorgensen K.A., Dyerberg J.: Antithrombin III and dietary intake of polyunsaturated fatty acids. Scand. J. Clin. Lab. Invest. 1982; 42: 83-86
14. Dyerberg J., Jorgensen K.A.: Marine oils and thrombogenesis. Progr. Lip. Res. 1982; 21: 255-269
15. Terano T., Hirai A., Hamazaki T., Kobayashi S., Fujita T., Tamura Y., Kumagai A.: Effect of oral administration of highly purified eicosapentaenoic acid on platelet function, blood viscosity and red cell deformability in healthy human subjects. Atherosclerosis 1983; 46: 321-331
16. Dehmer G.J., Popma J.J., van den Berg E.K., Eichhorn E.J., Prewitt J.B., Campbell W.B., Jennings L., Willerson J.T., Schmitz J.M.: Reduction in the rate of early restenosis after coronary angioplasty by a diet supplemented with n-3 fatty acids. New Engl. J. Med. 1988; 319:733-740
17. Lox C.D.: The effects of dietary marine fish oils (omega-3 fatty acids) on coagulation profiles in men. Gen. Pharmac. 1990; 21: 241-246
18. Muller A.D., van Houwelingen A.C., van Dam-Mieras M.C.E., Bas B.M., Hornstra G.: Effect of a moderate fish intake on haemostatic parameters in healthy males. Thromb. Haemost. 1989; 61: 468-473
19. Thorngren M., Gustafson A.: Effects of 11-week increase in dietary eicosapentaenoic acid on bleeding time, lipids and platelet aggregation. Lancet 1981; 2: 1190-1193
20. Yoshimura T, Matsui K., Yunohara T., Kawasaki N., Nakamura T., Okamura H.: Effects of highly purified eicosapentaenoic acid on plasma beta thromboglobulin level and vascular reactivity to angiotensin II. Artery 1987: 14: 295-303
21. Mortensen J.Z., Schmidt E.B., Nielsen A.H., Dyerberg J.: The effect of (n-6) and (n-3) polyunsaturated fatty acids on haemostasis, blood lipids and blood pressure. Thromb. Haemostas. 1983; 50: 543-546
22. Schmidt E.B., Kristensen S.D., Dyerberg J.: The effect of fish oil on lipids, coagulation and fibrinolysis in patients with angina pectoris. Artery 1988; 15: 316-329
23. Brox J.H., Killie J.E., Gunnes S., Nordoy A.: The effect of cod-liver oil and corn oil on platelets and vessel wall in man. Thromb. Haemostas. 1981; 46: 604-611
24. Brox J.H., Killie J.E., Østerud B., Holme S., Nordøy, A.: Effects of cod liver oil on platelets and coagulation in familial hypercholesterolemia (Type IIa). Acta Med. Scand. 1983; 213: 137-144
25. Rogers S., James K.S., Butland B.K., Etherington M.D., O'Brien J.R., Jones J.G.: Effects of a fish oil supplement on serum lipids, blood pressure, bleeding time, haemostatic and rheological variables. A double blind randomised controlled trial in healthy volunteers. Atherosclerosis 1987; 63: 137-143
26. Norris P.G., Jones C.J.H., Weston M.J.: Effect of dietary supplementation with fish oil on systolic blood pressure in mild essential hypertension. Brit. Med. J. 1986; 293: 104-105
27. Sanders T.A.B., Vickers M., Haines A.P.: Effect on blood lipids and haemostasis of a supplement of cod-liver oil, rich in eicosapentaenoic and docosahexaenoic acids, in healthy young men. Clin. Sci. 1981; 61: 317-324
28. Schmidt E.B., Ernst E., Varming K., Pedersen J.O., Dyerberg J.: The effect of n-3 fatty acids on lipids and haemostasis in patients with Type IIa and Type IV hyperlipidaemia. Thromb. Haemost. 1989; 62: 797-801
29. Schmidt E.B., Sorensen P.J., Pedersen J.O., Jersild C., Ditzel J., Grunnet N., Dyerberg J.: The effect of (n-3) polyunsaturated fatty acids on lipids, hemostasis, neutrophil and monocyte

chemotaxis in insulin dependent diabetes mellitus. J. Int. Med. 225 Suppl.1989; 1: 201-206

30. Haines A.P., Sanders T.A.B., Imeson J.D., Mahler R.F., Martin J., Mistry M., Vickers M., Wallace P.G.: Effects of a fish oil supplement on platelet function, hemostatic variables and albuminuria in insulin-dependent diabetics. Thromb. Res. 1986; 43: 643-655

31. Hostmark A.T., Bjerkedal T., Kierulf P., Flaten H., Ulshagen K.: Fish oil and plasma fibrinogen. Brit. Med. J. 1988; 297: 180-181

32. Radack K., Deck C., Huster G.: Dietary supplementation with low-dose fish oils lowers fibrinogen levels: a randomized. double-blind controlled study. Ann. Int. Med. 1989; 111: 757-758

33. Saynor R., Gillett T.: Fish oil and plasma fibrinogen. Brit. Med. J. 1988; 297: 1196

34. Hendra T.J., Britton M.E., Roper D.R., Wagaine-Twabwe D., Jeremy J.Y., Dandona P., Haines A.P., Yudkin J.S.: Effects of fish oil supplements in NIDDM subjects. Diabetes Care 1990; 13: 821-829

35. Green D., Barreres L., Borensztain J., Kaplan P., Reddy N., Rovner R., Simon H.: A double-blind, placebo-controlled trial of fish oil concentrate (MaxEPA) in stroke patients. Stroke 1985; 16: 706-709

36. Nordøy A., Lagarde M., Renaud S.: Platelets during alimentary hyperlipidaemia induced by cream and cod liver oil. Eur. J. Clin. Invest. 1984; 14

37. Dam-Mieras M.C.A., van Muller A.D., Rand M.L., Hornstra G.: Dietary lipids and macrophage procoagulant activity. Thrombosis Res. 1986; 43: 133-137

38. Hansen J.B., Olsen J.O., Wilsgard L., Østerud B.: Effects of dietary supplementation with cod liver oil on monocyte thromboplastin synthesis, coagulation and fibrinolysis. J. Int. Med. 225 Suppl. 1989; 1: 133-139

11. n-3 Fatty Acids and Fibrinolysis

E. B. Schmidt
Department of Medicine II, Aalborg Hospital, Denmark
(Department of Medicine, Section of Clinical Nutrition, Oregon Health Sciences University, Portland, Oregon, USA)

Fibrinolysis and Coronary Heart Disease

There is growing evidence[1-5] that an impairment of fibrinolysis increases the risk of coronary heart disease (CHD). Thus, fibrinolysis has been reported to be reduced in survivors of an acute myocardial infarction[1] and in patients with angiographically documented coronary atherosclerosis.[2]

Also, a depression of fibrinolysis seems to increase the risk for a recurrent myocardial infarction.[3]

Especially, increased levels in plasma of plasminogen activator inhibitor (PAI or PAI-1), the fast-acting inhibitor of tissue plasminogen activator in plasma, seem to increase the risk for CHD.[4,5]

The Effect of n-3 Fatty Acids on Fibrinolysis in Humans

The first study evaluating the effect of dietary n-3 fatty acids on fibrinolysis showed no effect of a daily supplement with 4 grams of n-3 fatty acids on euglobulin lysis time, considered an overall measure of fibrinolytic activity, when supplemented to 12 healthy males for a period of 6 weeks.[6]

Later, Barcelli and coworkers[7] reported that a daily supplement with 5 grams of n-3 fatty acids for 2 weeks significantly improved fibrinolysis by increasing levels of tissue plasminogen activator (t-PA) and by decreasing levels of PAI in plasma in 9 normal volunteers.

This study has been widely quoted, but unfortunately most other studies have shown either no effect or a reduction in fibrinolysis after ingestion of n-3 fatty acids.

Own Studies: Subjects and Methods

We have studied the effect of dietary supplementation with n-3 fatty acids on fibrinolysis in healthy subjects[8] and in patients with CHD[9] or at high risk for CHD, e.g. patients with insulin-dependent diabetes mellitus,[10] hyperlipidaemia[11] and hypertension.[12] We have determined t-PA antigen level, t-PA activity, and PAI (PAI-1) in plasma using commercially available test kits. Euglobulin lysis has been evaluated by the classical fibrin plate technique. Fibrinolysis has been determined at rest and in some of the studies after a short venous occlusion test (100 mm Hg; venous occlusion for 5 minutes).

Own Studies: Results

In general the most consistent finding in our studies has been the effect of supplementation with n-3 fatty acids on levels of PAI in plasma. The individual results of dietary supplementation with n-3 fatty acids on PAI in patients with CHD or at high risk for CHD are given in figure 1.

Each group of patients received from 4 to 6 grams of n-3 fatty acids per day for periods of 6-12 weeks as a supplement to their habitual diets. In most subjects and in most groups of subjects PAI levels increased (Fig. 1), although this was statistically significant only in patients with hypertension and type IIa hyperlipidaemia.

To study whether the apparent increase in levels of PAI in plasma depended on the dose of n-3 fatty acids given, we supplemented 10 healthy men for 6-week periods with 3 different daily doses of 1.3, 4, and 9 grams of n-3 fatty acids, respectively.[8] As shown in figure 2 there was a dose-dependent increase in PAI. Next, we were interested to study the effect of supplementation with n-3 fatty acids on levels of PAI when given for a longer period of time. Supplementation with 4 grams of n-3 fatty acids per day for 9 months to 24 healthy volunteers (14 women and 10 men; mean age 40 years; age range 21-53 years) resulted in a significant increase in PAI after 6 weeks of supplementation (Fig. 2). This increase was sustained, but not exaggerated, after 9 months of supplementation with n-3 fatty acids, also shown in figure 2.

We have also seen a non-significant increase in levels of PAI after daily supplementation with only 0.65 grams of n-3 fatty acids when given for 6 weeks (J. Moller et al. unpublished data). Finally, we have recently completed a study where 20 healthy volunteers were given 20 g of n-3 fatty acids as a single dose with their evening meal. PAI was measured 14 hours later at 8am and compared to values obtained at 8am before the supplement. PAI levels significantly increased after this very high intake of n-3 fatty acids (J. Moller et al. unpublished data).

In our studies no consistent effect of dietary supplementation with n-3 fatty acids on levels of t-PA antigen or t-PA activity has emerged. However, some of the results

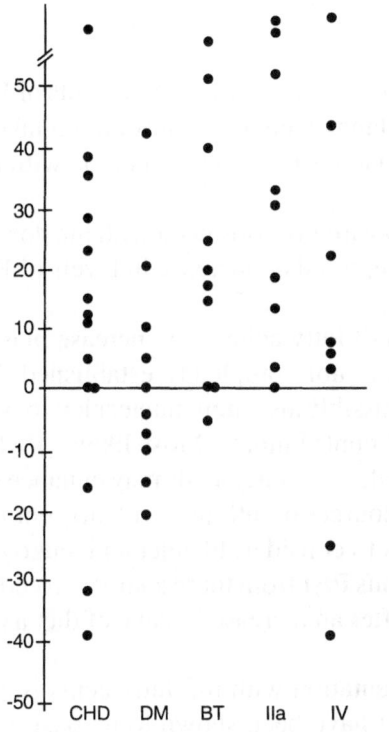

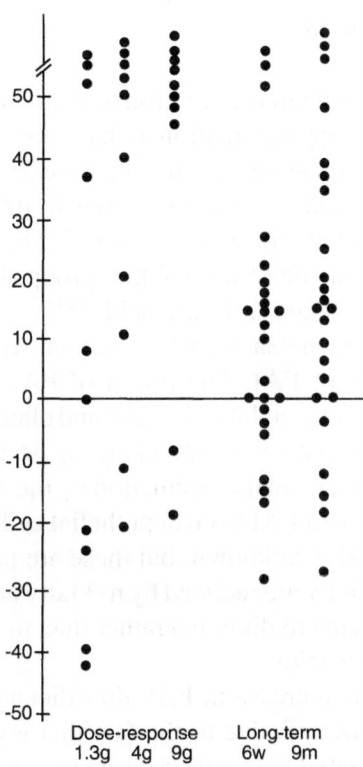

Fig. 1. The percent change in plasma levels of PAI after dietary supplementation with n-3 fatty acids is shown for individual patients.
Abbreviations: CHD = coronary heart disease, DM = insulin-dependent diabetes mellitus, BT = hypertension, IIa and IV = patients with type IIa and type IV hyperlipidaemia, respectively.

Fig. 2. The percent change in plasma levels of PAI after supplementation with n-3 fatty acids is shown for individual subjects. Individual results are given for the dose-response study after 6 weeks of supplementation with 1.3, 4 and 9 grams of n-3 fatty acids per day, respectively (left). Individual data for subjects in the long-term study are given after 6 weeks and 9 months of supplementation with n-3 fatty acids (right).

should be briefly considered. Thus euglobulin lysis time was reduced in patients with angina pectoris after 12 weeks of supplementation with 4.5 grams of n-3 fatty acids per day.[9] A depression of fibrinolysis may be of particular concern in these patients with a high risk of future coronary events. Finally, t-PA activity was markedly reduced both at rest and after a short venous occlusion test in patients with hyperlipidaemia after 6 weeks of supplementation with 6 grams of n-3 fatty acids per day.[11]

Discussion

The main finding from our studies has been an increase in plasma levels of PAI after supplementation with n-3 fatty acids. PAI may increase rapidly after intake of n-3 fatty acids, and the increase seems to persist during supplementation with n-3 fatty acids for longer periods of time.

Finally, the increase in PAI is likely to be positively correlated with the dose of n-3 fatty acids used. Other groups have also reported an increase in levels of PAI after dietary n-3 fatty acids.[13,14]

It is unclear by what mechanisms dietary n-3 fatty acids may increase plasma levels of PAI. The origin of PAI in plasma is not completely established, but especially endothelial cells and platelets, and possibly also mononuclear leukocytes and hepatocytes are likely to be significant contributors.[5] Most likely, PAI is cleared from the circulation by the liver.[5] Whether n-3 fatty acids may enhance the release of PAI from endothelial cells or other sources or interfere with the removal of PAI is unknown, but these are possibilities to consider. Platelet and leukocyte reactivity are reduced by n-3 fatty acids, and thus PAI from these sources would be expected to diminish rather than to increase after an increased intake of dietary n-3 fatty acids.

The increase in PAI after dietary supplementation with n-3 fatty acids is also unexpected, due to the fact that levels of PAI have been shown to be positively correlated to triglycerides in plasma by several investigators.[1,4] Therefore, dietary supplementation with n-3 fatty acids, which consistently (and also in our aforementioned studies) has been shown to reduce triglycerides in plasma, would be expected to decrease levels of PAI.

Furthermore, very low-density-lipoproteins have recently been reported to enhance the release of PAI from human endothelial cells in culture,[4] and the secretion of very low-density-lipoproteins is reduced by n-3 fatty acids. Still unexplained and unexpected, the increase in PAI after dietary n-3 fatty acids is, however, in line with higher plasma levels of PAI in Greenland Eskimos than in matched controls.[15]

Studies elucidating the mechanisms by which dietary n-3 fatty acids may affect fibrinolysis are clearly warranted.

Conclusion

Dietary n-3 fatty acids may impair fibrinolysis by increasing levels of PAI in plasma. The mechanisms operating are unknown. This untoward effect of n-3 fatty acids should not be seen in isolation but viewed in the light of a multiplicity of beneficial effects exerted by n-3 fatty acids with respect to atherosclerosis and thrombosis, as indicated by other presentations in this book.

References

1. Hamsten A., Wiman B., De Faire U., Blomback M.: Increased plasma levels of tissue plasminogen activator in young survivors of myocardial infarction. N. Engl. J. Med. 1985; 313: 1557-1563

2. Francis R.B., Kawanishi D., Baruch T., Mahrer P., Rahimtoola S., Feinstein D.I.: Impaired fibrinolysis in coronary artery disease. Am. Heart J. 1988; 115: 776-780

3. Hamsten A., Walldius G., Szamosi A., Blomback M., De Faire U., Dahlen G., Wiman B.: Plasminogen activator inhibitor in plasma: risk factor for recurrent myocardial infarction. Lancet 1987; 2:3-9

4. Stiko-Rahm A., Wiman B., Hamsten A., Nilsson J.: Secretion of plasminogen activator inhibitor-1 from cultured human umbilical vein endothelial cells is induced by very low density lipoprotein. Arteriosclerosis 1990; 10: 1067-1073

5. Kruithof E.K.O.: Plasminogen activator inhibitor 1: Biochemical, biological and clinical aspects. Fibrinolysis 1988; 2 (suppl 2): 59-70

6. Sanders T.A.B., Vickers M., Haines A.P.: Effect on blood lipids and haemostasis of a supplement of cod-liver oil, rich in eicosapentaenoic and docosahexaenoic acids, in healthy young men. Clinical Science 1981; 61: 317-324.

7. Barcelli U., Glas-Greenwalt P., Pollak V.E.: Enhancing effect of dietary supplementation with n-3 fatty acids on plasma fibrinolysis in normal subjects. Thromb. Res. 1985; 39: 307-312

8. Schmidt E.B., Varming K., Ernst E., Madsen P., Dyerberg J.: Dose-response studies on the effect of n-3 polyunsaturated fatty acids on lipids and haemostasis. Thromb. Haemostas. 1990; 63: 1-5

9. Schmidt E.B., Kristensen S.D., Dyerberg J.: The effect of fish oil on lipids, coagulation and fibrinolysis in patients with stable angina pectoris. Artery 1988; 15: 316-329

10. Schmidt E.B., Sorensen P.J., Pedersen J.O., Jersild C., Ditzel J., Grunnet N., Dyerberg J.: The effect of n-3 polyunsaturated fatty acids on lipids, haemostasis, neutrophil and monocyte chemotaxis in insulin-dependent diabetes mellitus. J. Intern. Med. 1989; 225 (suppl 1): 201-206

11. Schmidt E.B., Ernst E., Varming K., Pedersen J.O., Dyerberg J.: The effect of n-3 fatty acids on lipids and haemostasis in patients with type IIa and type IV hyperlipidaemia. Thromb. Haemostas. 1989; 62: 797-801

12. Schmidt E.B., Nielsen L.K., Pedersen J.O., Kornerup H.J., Dyerberg J.: The effect of n-3 polyunsaturated fatty acids on lipids, platelet function, coagulation, fibrinolysis and monocyte chemotaxis in patients with hypertension. Clin. Chim. Acta 1990; 189: 25-32

13. Emeis J.J., van Houwelingen A.C., van den Hoogen C.M., Hornstra G.: A moderate fish intake increases plasminogen activator inhibitor type-1 in human volunteers. Blood 1989; 74: 233-237

14. Froschl H., Spannagl M., Drummer C., Landgraf-Leurs MMC., Landgraf R., Schramm W.: Effect of eicosapentaenoic acid diet on humoral clotting and fibrinolysis parameters in Type I diabetes mellitus. Haemostasis 1988; 18 (suppl 2): 27-28

15. Schmidt E.B., Sorensen P.J., Ernst E., Kristensen S.D., Pedersen J.O., Dyerberg J.: Studies on coagulation and fibrinolysis in Greenland Eskimos. Thromb. Res. 1989; 56: 553-55

12. Effects of n-3 Fatty Acids on Monocyte Functions

E. Tremoli, E. Stragliotto, S. Colli, S. Eligini, C. Mosconi, P. Maderna, C. Galli

Institute of Pharmacological Sciences and E. Grossi Paoletti Center, University of Milan, Italy

The accumulation of lipid laden macrophages into the vasculature is one of the early events in the development of atherosclerosis. Monocytes/macrophages display a number of features which are thought to play a role in thrombosis and atherosclerosis. Indeed, these cells are able to contribute to these processes by means of their secretory products, such as O_2^- derived cytotoxic compounds, biologically active metabolites of arachidonic acid, platelet activating factor (PAF), and cytokines. They may also display procoagulant and both pro- and anti-fibrinolytic activities.[1]

In the past few years it has been demonstrated that n-3 fatty acids may interfere at various levels with monocyte/macrophage functions, as demonstrated by a number of recently published studies. They have been shown indeed to inhibit generation of leukotrienes,[2] monocyte chemotaxis[3] and synthesis of interleukin 1 and of tumor necrosis factor (TNF).[4]

Recently Østerud et al. have shown that n-3 fatty acid administration to humans reduces the expression of procoagulant activity (PCA) of mononuclear cells.[5] In a recent study we evaluated the effects of the administration of EPA and DHA ethyl ester preparations in healthy male volunteers. The subjects were given for 6 weeks 6 capsules/day of the K85 preparation (Norsk Hydro, Norway) each capsule containing 465 mg EPA and 283 mg DHA for a total of 2.8 and 1.7 g of EPA and DHA respectively. During treatment the subjects received vitamin E (Ephynal, Roche) supplementation, 300 mg every other day. At baseline and after 6 weeks of administration, fatty acid composition in cell membranes of various cell types was monitored.[6,7] Concomitantly, platelet function, i.e. aggregation evaluated by

Table I. Fatty acid composition of platelet, PMN and monocyte lipids.

Fatty acids	Platelets		PMN		Monocytes	
	Time 0	6 weeks	Time 0	6 weeks	Time 0	6 weeks
18:2 n-6	6.3 ±0.27	6.1 ±0.33	10.2 ±0.73	9.1 ±0.6	8.9 ±0.37	9.1 ±0.45
20:4 n-6	22.8 ±0.35	19.8 ±0.6**	10.2 ±0.57	7.6 ±0.26**	15.3 ±0.75	11.3 ±0.61**
20:5 n-3	0.34±0.06	1.88±0.1*	0.43±0.07	1.25±0.05*	0.26±0.02	1.14±0.08*
22:6 n-3	0.87±0.12	1.13±0.16	0.48±0.1	1.27±0.19**	1.34±0.09	1.84±0.17***

Values are expressed as weight percentages, as averages ± SEM (n=5 subjects).
The values with the asterisk are significantly different from values before treatment at the following levels:
* $p < 0.001$; ** $p < 0.01$; *** $p < 0.05$

Born's method, the synthesis of thromboxane B_2 and the levels of ^{3}H-labelled inositol phosphates following stimulation of platelets with thrombin were studied.[8-10] Mononuclear cell and neutrophil functions were also evaluated. Neutrophils were obtained from blood by conventional methods[11] and monocytes were isolated by adherence to plastic starting from the mononuclear cell preparation.[12] Purity of adherent monocytes was >90% as defined by cytochemical reactivity for α-naphthylacetate esterase.[13] Superoxide anion generation by neutrophils and adherent monocytes was determined according to Babior.[14] Basal or LPS-stimulated PCA was assayed in adherent monocytes.[15]

In platelets, accumulation of EPA and DHA was accompanied by changes in the levels of n-6 fatty acids, with an increase in linoleic acid content and a significant decrease in arachidonic acid (Tab. I). These changes resulted in a significant increase in the concentrations of collagen necessary to induce "in vitro" 50% of maximal aggregation, and in a marked (>50%) inhibition in thromboxane generation by platelets in response to 5 U/ml thrombin or 5 μg/ml collagen. These platelet effects were accompanied by reductions in inositol phosphate levels, measured by the generation of inositol monophosphate, bisphosphate and tris-phosphate from ^{3}H-myo-inositol-labelled platelets; such a reduction after the 6th week of n-3 fatty acid supplementation was more prominent in the unstimulated condition, but also detected in thrombin-stimulated cells (data not shown).

In monocyte/macrophages, concomitant with the increase in n-3 fatty acid content of cell membranes (Tab. I) was the reduction in the generation of superoxide anion after stimulation of cells with different agonists (Fig. 1). This effect was not due to the partial depletion in the arachidonic acid content of the monocytes, because arachidonic acid *in vitro* added to monocytes failed to correct the impairment in the generation of superoxide anion induced by the treatment by

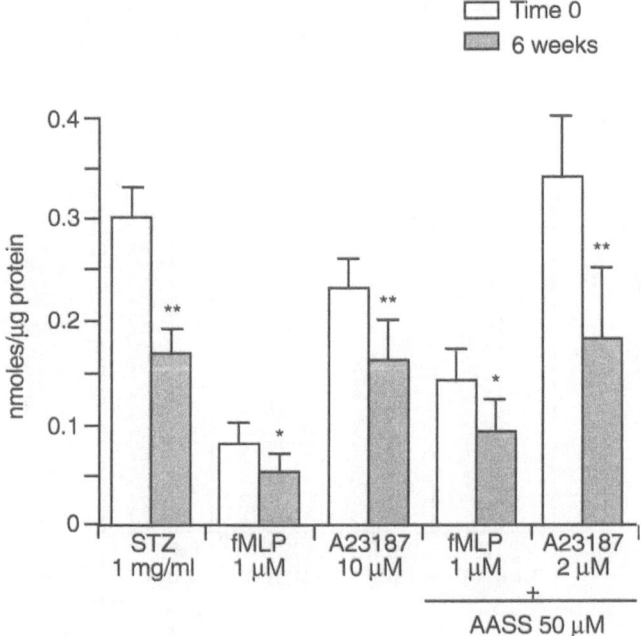

Fig. 1. Effect of n-3 fatty acid ethylesters, given for 6 weeks to healthy volunteers, on the superoxide anion generation by monocytes. STZ: serum treated zymosan; fMLP: formyl-methionyl-leucyl-phenyl-alanine. AASS: arachidonic acid sodium salt; * p<0.05; ** p<0.02

n-3 fatty acids. In addition to that, it should be noted that a similar reduction in the arachidonic acid content in membranes was present in both monocytes and neutrophils; in these last cells, however, there was no significant effect of n-3 fatty acids on the generation of O_2^- (Fig. 2). Interestingly, a reduction in the production of superoxide anion could be detected using a more complex method evaluating the production of superoxide anion by the leukocytes present in whole blood, after the treatment with n-3 fatty acids (data not shown).

The effects of n-3 fatty acids on the monocyte capacity to express PCA was also evaluated, in the same set of experiments, both before and after stimulation of adherent monocytes with bacterial lipopolysaccharide (Fig. 3). In both experimental conditions, a reduction in procoagulant activity could be demonstrated.

The evidence discussed above indicates that oral administration of n-3 fatty acid ethylesters influences the response of monocyte/macrophages to the effects of specific agonists. The accumulation of n-3 fatty acids in plasma membranes of human monocytes induces a significant impairment in the capacity of these cells to produce cytotoxic species and localize fibrin formation through the expression of procoagulant activity. These effects may be of particular relevance in the athero-sclerotic process. In fact, free radicals and superoxide anion have been recently

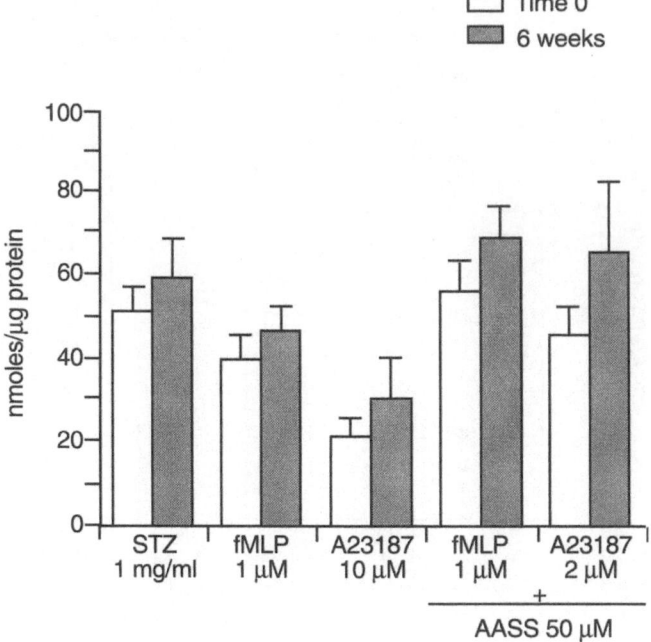

Fig. 2. Effect of n-3 fatty acid ethylesters, given for 6 weeks to healthy volunteers, on the superoxide anion generation by PMN. Note that, at variance with monocytes, there is no detectable effect. Abbreviations as in Fig. 1.

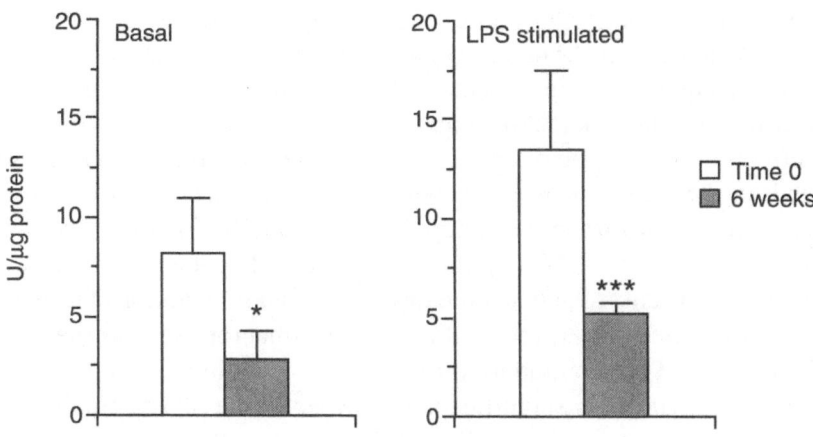

Fig. 3. Effects of n-3 fatty acids on expression of procoagulant activity (PCA) by monocytes. LPS: bacterial lipopolysaccharide. * $p < 0.05$; ** $p < 0.001$

considered to be causally involved in low density lipoprotein (LDL) modifications, leading to the generation of oxidized or minimally modified LDL which are claimed to possess a greater atherosclerotic potential with respect to native LDL.[16] On the other hand, procoagulant activity of monocyte/ macrophages may be of relevance in order to localize fibrin formation in the vessel wall.[17] Indeed it is known that monocytes are the first cells adhering to undamaged endothelium during experimental atherosclerosis.[18]

Therefore the capacity of n-3 fatty acids to reduce the generation of both superoxide anion and procoagulant activity by human monocytes appears promising for the overall evaluation of the potential antiatherosclerotic effects of n-3 fatty acids. The relevance, however, of these changes of monocyte function in the overall processes of thrombosis and atherosclerosis remains to be defined.

References

1. Wissler R.W., Vesselinovitch D., Davis H.R. In: Olsson A.G. (Ed) *Atherosclerosis: Biology and Clinical Science.* New York: Churchill Livingstone 1987 p. 57
2. Lee T.H., Hoover R.L., Williams J.D., Sperling R.I., Ravalese J. III, Spur B.W., Robinson D.R., Corey E.J., Lewis R.A., Austen K.F.: Effect of dietary enrichment with eicosapentaenoic and docosahexaenoic acids on in vitro neutrophil and monocyte leukotriene generation and neutrophil function. New Engl. J. Med. 1985; 312: 1217-1224
3. Schmidt E.B., Pedersen J.O., Ekelund S., Grunnet N., Jersild C., Dyerberg J.: Cod liver oil inhibits neutrophil and monocyte chemotaxis in healthy males. Atherosclerosis 1989; 77 :53-57
4. Endres S., Ghorbani R., Kelley V.E., Georgilis K., Lonnemann G., van der Meer J.W.M., Cannon J.G., Rogers T.S., Klempner M.S., Werber P.C., Schaefer E.J., Wolff S.M., Dinarello C.A.: The effects of dietary supplementation with n-3 polyunsaturated fatty acids on the synthesis of interleukin-1 and tumor necrosis factor by mononuclear cells. New Engl. J. Med. 1989; 2320: 265-271
5. Hansen J.B., Olsen J.O., Wilsgard L., Osterud B.: Effects of dietary supplementation with cod liver oil on monocyte thromboplastin synthesis, coagulation and fibrinolysis. J. Int. Med. 1989; 225 731 (suppl.): 133-139
6. Folch J., Lees M., Sloan-Stanley G.H. A simple method for the isolation and purification of total lipides from animal tissues J. Biol. Chem. 1957; 226: 497-509
7. Rouser G, Kritchevsky G, Yamamoto A, Simon G, Galli C, Bauman AJ. In: Lowenstein JM (ed.) *Lipids. Methods in Enzymology Vol. 14.* New York, Academic Press 1969; 272
8. Born GVR: Aggregation of blood platelets by adenosine diphosphate and its reversal. Nature 1962; 194: 927-929
9. Tremoli E, Maderna P, Colli S, Morazzoni G, Sirtori M, Sirtori CR.: Increased platelet sensitivity and thromboxane b_2 formation in type-II hyperlipoproteinaemic patients. Eur. J. Clin. Invest. 1984; 14: 329-333
10. Berridge MJ.: Rapid accumulation of inositol trisphosphate reveals that agonists hydrolyse polyphosphoinositides instead of phosphatidylinositol. Biochem. J. 1983; 212, 3: 849-58
11. Böyum A.: Isolation of leucocytes from human blood. Further observations. Methylcellulose, dextran, and ficoll as erythrocyte aggregating agents. Scand. J. Clin. Lab. Invest. 1968, 21, suppl. 97: 31-50

12. Fisher DG, Karen HS. *Methods for studying mononuclear phagocytes.* New York, Academic Press Inc. 1981; 4347

13. Li CY, Lam KW, Yam LT.: Esterases in human leucocytes. J. Histochem. Cytochem. 1973; 21: 1-12

14. Babior BM, Kipnes RS, Curnutte JT.: Biological defense mechanisms. The production by leucocytes of superoxide, a potential bactericidal agent. J. Clin. Invest. 1973; 51: 741-44

15. Rambaldi A, Alessio G, Casali B, Gambacorti Passerini C, Donati MB, Mantovani A, Semeraro N.: Induction of monocyte-macrophage procoagulant activity by transformed cell lines. J. Immunol. 1986; 136: 3848-55

16. Steinberg D, Parthasarathy S, Carew TE, Khoo JC, Witztum JL.: Beyond cholesterol. Modifications of low-density lipoprotein that increase its atherogenicity. New Engl. J. Med. 1989; 320: 915-924

17. Gimbrone M.A. In: Gimbrone MA (Ed.) *Vascular endothelium in hemostasis and thrombosis.* 1986; 1

18. Faggiotto A, Ross R.: Studies of hypercholesterolemia in the non human primate I. Changes that lead to fatty streak formation: II. Fatty streak conversion to fibrous plaque. Arteriosclerosis 1984; 4, 4: 323-340; 341-356

13. Prevention of Cardiac Arrhythmias by n-3 Fatty Acids

H. HALLAQ, A. LEAF

Medical Services, Massachusetts General Hospital, Boston, Massachusetts, USA

The recently published DART study showed that ingesting fatty fish two or three times weekly by male subjects following a myocardial infarction was associated with a reduction in total mortality from heart attacks but not in the incidence of infarction.[1] These results suggest that the beneficial effect of n-3 fatty acids may be mediated by preventing arrhythmias ensuing during acute myocardial ischemia - the major cause of death from heart attacks. Indeed, it had been shown already in experimental myocardial infarction in rats that different dietary interventions may have dramatic effects on arrhythmias occurring during ischemia and/or reperfusion. A diet high in saturated fat was associated with an increased incidence and duration of ventricular fibrillation during ischemia as well as during post-ischemic reperfusion of the coronary arteries. A diet rich in sunflower seed oil had a moderate protective effect, whereas a diet enriched with tuna fish oil, with a high content of the long chain polyunsaturated n-3 fatty acids (n-3 PUFAs) EPA and DHA, was associated with a very significant reduction in ventricular fibrillation, especially in older animals.[2]

To learn more about the possible mechanism of protection from serious arrhythmias we have undertaken studies on another very reproducible form of cardiac arrhythmias, namely that induced by toxic levels of the digitalis glycoside ouabain. Our experimental preparation has been isolated neonatal rat cardiac myocytes. This seems an ideal tissue for such studies as the cells from the neonatal rat heart, when separated into individual cells, beat spontaneously and regularly for several days in culture media.

We can thus measure the amplitude of contraction and the beating rate of individual cells and examine the effects of various agents on these parameters of function in the absence of hemodynamic or neurohumoral factors.

The administration of a toxic concentration of ouabain (10^{-4} M) to the medium bathing these cells causes an increased beating rate, contracture and grossly irregular rhythm (the *in vitro* equivalent of fibrillation).

This ouabain toxicity is not modified by pretreatment of the myocytes with arachidonic acid (C20:4n-6; AA), but it is completely prevented by addition of 2

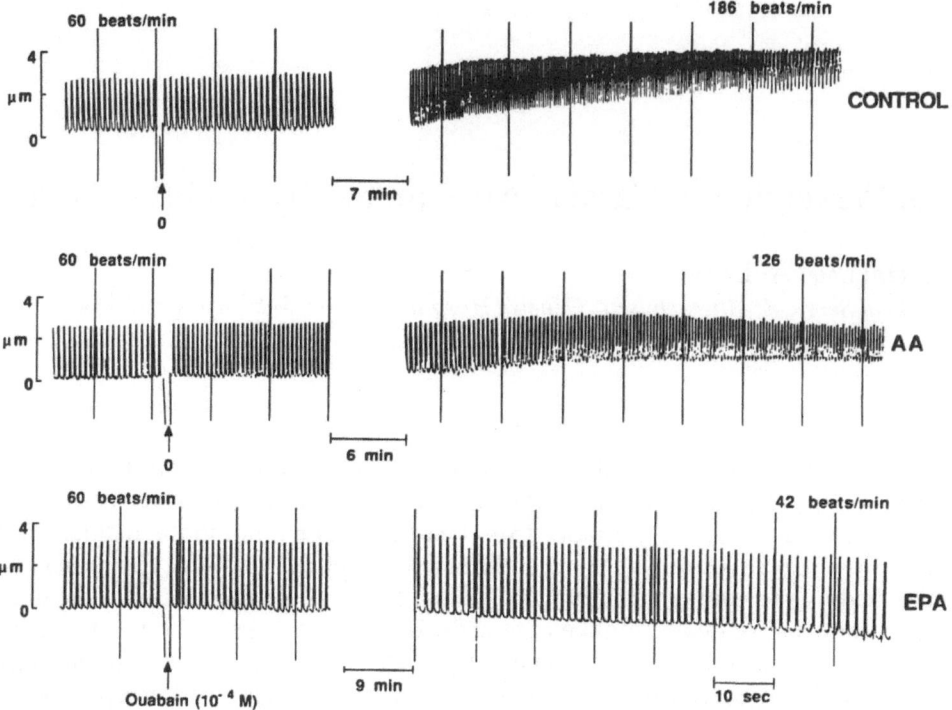

Fig. 1. The effect of 0.1 mM ouabain on the contractile state of single representative cardiac myocytes incubated 3 to 5 days without supplementary fatty acids added to the incubating medium (top tracing) or with arachidonic acid (AA; middle tracing) or with eicosapentaenoic acid (EPA; bottom tracing) present in the incubating medium. The toxic effects of ouabain are seen in the control and AA-enriched myocytes as an increased rate and a decreased amplitude of contractions as the myocytes proceed to contracture. The irregular amplitude of beats at the end of the control tracing is the *in vitro* equivalent of fibrillation. By contrast, the toxic effects were not exhibited by the EPA-enriched myocytes, as seen in the bottom tracing. (From ref. 3 with permission of the publisher)

to 5 μM of eicosapentaenoic acid (C20:5n-3; EPA) to the medium bathing the cells. Representative results are shown in figure 1 and the summary findings, in table I. Docosahexaenoic acid (C22:6n-3; DHA) affords protection similar to EPA. Furthermore, the protection afforded by these two n-3 PUFA can be fully achieved when the fatty acids are added together with the ouabain, indicating that incorporation of these n-3 fatty acids in cellular membranes is not of importance in the protective effect. To determine the mechanism of this protective action of the n-3 PUFA the possibility that they were somehow interfering with the inhibition by ouabain of the Na,K-ATPase of the cardiac myocytes was examined. When the activity of the Na,K-ATPase was assayed in cells exposed to 0 or to 10^{-4} or 10^{-3} M ouabain, there was no effect of EPA or DHA on the degree of inhibition of this enzyme, which is the only known site of action of ouabain. Since calcium is essential for contraction of muscle cells, the level of cytosolic free calcium was determined using the fluorescent indicator fura-2. Here a definite effect was

Table I. Changes in amplitude of contraction and beating rate of neonatal rat cardiac myocytes produced by 0.1 mM oubain. Measurements of beating rate and of amplitude of contractions were made just prior to and 6 to 9 minutes after exposure to 0.1 mM ouabain.

Media addition	Amplitude (μm)		Beats/min	
	control	ouabain (10⁻⁴ M)	control	ouabain (10⁻⁴ M)
none	2.76±0.1	1.50±0.19	72±3.6	165±16
(n)	(6)	(6)	(6)	(6)
AA	2.81±0.24	1.35±0.12	71±2.5	161±16
(n)	(4)	(4)	(4)	(4)
EPA	2.88±0.13	3.84±0.14	80±4.0	55±4
(n)	(6)	(6)	(6)	(6)

Values are means ± SEM. AA = arachidonic acid, 5 μM, in incubation media for 3 to 5 days. EPA = eicosapentaenoic acid, 5 μM, in incubation media for 3 to 5 days.
Numbers in parentheses are n. (From ref. 3 with permission of the publisher).

observed as the EPA prevented the rise in cytosolic calcium to toxic levels, as shown in table II. This would protect the myocytes from the contracture and arrhythmias that characterize the toxic effects of ouabain. When calcium influx into the myocytes was measured with $^{45}Ca^{2+}$, it was found that both EPA and DHA inhibited the influx of calcium in the presence of ouabain by some 30 percent[4] and that this blockage of calcium influx must at least contribute to the protective action of these n-3 PUFA from fish oils against the toxic effects of high concentrations of ouabain on the cardiac myocytes. Thus these fatty acids appeared to be acting as calcium channel blockers. Further studies have now shown[4] that the action of these fatty acids is not as simple calcium channel blockers but that they modulate the dihydropyridine sensitive calcium channels in the sarcolemma of these cardiac myocytes. The basis for this statement is that when the calcium channel agonist, the

Table II. Changes in cytosolic free calcium, $[Ca^{2+}]_i$ induced by ouabain. $[Ca^{2+}]_i$ was measured in neonatal rat cardiac myocytes incubated with ouabain at 0, 1 μM, or 0.1 mM using fura-2.

Media addition	[0M]	Ouabain [10⁻⁶M]	[10⁻⁴M]
None	143±11	294±59	845±29
(n)	(8)	(3)	(5)
AA	147±11	329±29	757±64
(n)	(7)	(3)	(5)
EPA	141±10	227±2	214±16
(n)	(8)	(3)	(5)

Values are mean ± SEM. AA (5 μM) or EPA (5 μM)were added to the incubation medium for 3 to 5 days.
$[Ca^{2+}]_i$ measurements were made just prior to and 9 to 11 minutes after exposure of the cells to ouabain.
(From ref. 3 with permission of the publisher).

88

dihydropyridine Bay K8644 (10^{-6} M), was added to the myocytes it increased the calcium influx and caused contracture of the cells similar to the changes induced by ouabain. Addition of EPA or DHA (2 to 5 µM) with the Bay K 8644 blocked the increased calcium influx and prevented cell contracture.

However, addition of nitrendipine (10^{-9} M), a dihydropyridine calcium channel antagonist, to these cells stops their contractions completely and in "diastole" because insufficient calcium enters the cells to sustain contractility. When the n-3 PUFAs were added with nitrendipine they prevented the inhibitory effect of nitrendipine on these cells. Thus these n-3 PUFAs can inhibit excess calcium entry into the cardiac myocytes when too much calcium is entering the cells, as occurs with ouabain toxicity or Bay K8644 stimulation. But they can also open the L-type calcium channels and thus sustain normal myocyte contractility when insufficient calcium is entering the cells, as following exposure to the calcium channel blocker, nitrendipine. Thus the fish oil fatty acids can exert a dual effect on calcium transport; they can prevent excessive calcium influx and they can enhance insufficient calcium influx when either extreme threatens to compromise the functional integrity of the cardiac myocyte. Finally these modulatory effects of the n-3 fatty acids are apparently specific for the dihydropyridine-sensitive calcium channels and somehow affect only the dihydropyridine site on these calcium channels. Thus, determination of ^{3}H-nitrendipine binding to the cardiac myocytes in the presence and absence of n-3 fatty acids indicates non-competitive inhibition of nitrendipine binding in the presence of n-3 PUFA. When the same L-type calcium channels are blocked by verapamil or diltiazem, which are known to affect the calcium channels by binding at some sites largely independent of the dihydropyridine binding sites, the n-3 PUFA are incapable of preventing the blocking of the calcium channels induced by these agents. These studies indicate a role for the long-chain n-3 polyunsaturated fatty acids in the regulation of cardiac contractility through modulation of calcium channels in cardiac myocytes. Fish and fish oils are the primary sources of these fatty acids in our diets. Modest dietary modifications may affect the function of our hearts in health and disease, but much remains to be tested.

Acknowledgements The studies reported were supported in part by National Institutes of Health Grants DK38165, HL40548, and P50 DK39249.
We thank Dr. Thomas W. Smith for generously making available instruments essential for this research.

References

1. Burr, L. M., Gilbert, F. J., Holliday, M. R., Elwood, P. C., Fehily, M. A., Rogers, S., Sweetnam, M. P., Deadman, M. N.: Effects of changes in fat, fish, and fibre intakes on death and myocardial reinfarction: diet and reinfarction trial (DART) Lancet 1989; 2 (8666): 757-761
2. McLennan, P. L., Abeywardena, M.Y., Charnock, J. S.: Dietary fish oil prevents ventricular fibrillation following coronary artery occlusion and reperfusion. Can. J. Physiol. Pharmacol. 1985; 63: 1441-47; Am. Heart J. 1988; 116 (3): 709-717
3. Hallaq, H., Sellmayer, A., Smith, T. W., Leaf, A.: Protective effect of eicosapentaenoic acid on ouabain toxicity in neonatal rat cardiac myocytes. Proc. Natl. Acad. Sci. USA 1990; 87 (20): 7834-38
4. Hallaq H., Smith T.W., Leaf, A. Proc. Natl. Acad. Sci. USA, 1991 In press.

n-3 Fatty Acids and Hypertension

14. Essential Hypertension: Current Needs and Methodological Problems with Non-pharmacological Treatment

P.R. JACKSON, W.W. YEO, L.E. RAMSAY

University Department of Medicine and Therapeutics, Royal Hallamshire Hospital, Sheffield, UK

Epidemiological studies have shown that a significant proportion of the population have diastolic blood pressures above 100 mmHg even on rechecking. Trials from many countries demonstrate that treatment of such patients with hypotensive drugs reduces the risk of stroke, heart failure and renal failure.[1,2,3,4] The benefit in terms of a reduced risk of myocardial infarction is smaller but an overview of the trials shows that even this disorder may be reduced by about 14%.[5] Thus, the detection and treatment of people with high blood pressure represents one of the major challenges in the prevention of cardiovascular disease. Reduction in blood pressure may be achieved by means other than drug treatment such as weight loss, restricting excess alcohol intake and cutting back on salt consumption. Further benefit may be gained by getting patients to quit smoking thus preventing added cardiovascular damage. In normal practice pharmacological treatment would only be initiated if the blood pressure remains elevated despite such measures.

When assessing new treatments for the control of hypertension physicians require good evidence, not only of therapeutic benefit but also of any adverse effects produced by therapy. Commonly a slightly lower burden of proof has been required when studying the efficacy of non-pharmacological therapy and such interventions have often been assumed to be unlikely to produce adverse effects. Thus, the advice to reduce salt consumption is based on epidemiological studies[6] and a series of trials which show conflicting results, the largest showing no effect.[7] The doses of n-3 polyunsaturated fatty acids (PUFA) advised in hypertension are clearly pharmacological rather than physiological and I believe such agents should not be exempt from the rigorous examination to which other pharmacological agents are subjected. We need, therefore, to obtain data on their efficacy not only

Table I. Limitations of uncontrolled observations and ways for their overcoming

•**Observer bias**	- Blind
•**Patient bias**	- Blind
•**Change in disease with time**	- Control group
•**Bias in treatment allocation**	- Randomize
•**"Soft" end-points**	- Standardize
•**Altered compliance**	- Monitor
•**Groups dissimilar by chance**	- Stratify
•**Placebo effect**	- Control group
•**Regression to the mean**	- Control group
•**Response observed by chance**	- Statistics

Table II. Controlled trial

•**Double blind**
•**Controlled:** *vs* placebo or standard treatment
•**Well-designed:** parallel group or crossover
•**Random** (stratified/minimization?)
•**Groups similar**
•**Standard end-points**
•**Adequate power**
•**Compliance monitored**
•**Properly analysed**

from uncontrolled observations (epidemiological evidence or uncontrolled clinical trials), but also from controlled clinical trials.

The reason that uncontrolled observations alone do not warrant sufficient weight of evidence is their numerous limitations. These deficiencies are set out in table I along with strategies to overcome them. Generally a good controlled trial will contain these along with other features to protect the study from generating a spurious outcome (Tab. II).

The fundamental importance of a control group within a clinical trial is highlighted by the observations that placebo is able treat 25% of peptic ulcers, to control blood pressure in 30% of the patients and to cure 100% of patients with common cold. These findings are either due to the natural history of the disease studied or to regression towards the mean. Only when a control group is included in a study may the true effect of the treatment be isolated. If a treatment of proven efficacy versus placebo is already available, comparison with this rather than placebo is an acceptable alternative and may be superior when placebo treatment is difficult to justify ethically. Here, the choice of such a standard can introduce bias as has been seen with comparisons of novel hypotensive drugs with methyl-dopa which has tended to emphasize the relative lack of adverse effects of the new agent. Choice of placebo is not simple when investigating PUFA as the distinctive taste of marine oil makes blinding of patients to the treatments difficult. Rather than choosing other oils which still may be differentiated by taste from marine oils and could have their own pharmacological effects it would perhaps be best to abandon patient blinding and explore other strategies to avoid patient bias. One would be to explain to patients that the study involves two active agents and mention the marine source of one at the outset. The comparative treatment could then be a standard treatment or still placebo which would be ethically justifiable as blood pressure is known to fall during at least four months of placebo therapy.[2] Care must be taken to maintain blinding of the investigator and this would require separation of the blood pressure measuring and adverse effect detecting functions, lest the complaint of fishy breath reveal to the investigator recording the blood pressure which treatment the patient is receiving. Blinding of investigators is of key importance because even random zero sphygmomanometers do not completely exclude digit preference and worse practices.

Two clinical trials designs are widely used; the parallel group and the cross-over designs (Fig. 1). The parallel group study is amenable to straightforward statistical analysis and its duration is unlimited, which can be helpful when effects are slow to appear. The main disadvantage of this study design is variability between individuals which inflates the variance of the estimated treatment effect. A large

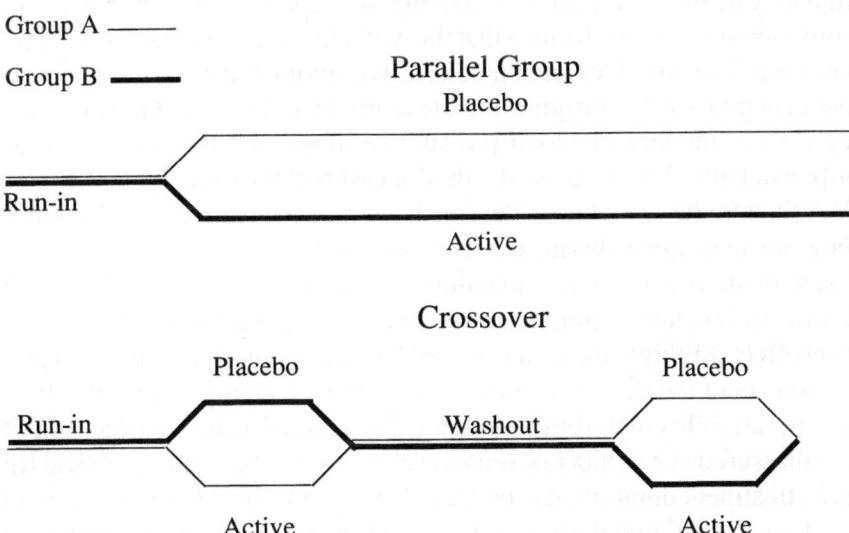

Fig. 1. Parallel group and crossover trial designs.

sample size is therefore required to achieve statistical significance if the size of the effect is moderate or small. Poor randomization, leading to marked imbalance between the groups, may well exacerbate this problem. In the cross-over design variability between patients is no longer a problem since each subject receives both treatments but in a randomized sequence. However, its duration is inevitably limited and there is the possible confounding effect of treatment-period interaction (carry-over effect). This latter effect may be of importance in studying the effects of n-3 PUFA, since it has been shown that concentrations of important biological mediators like interleukin I and tumour necrosis factor are reduced by n-3 PUFA treatment, and that this effect lasts for up to 10 weeks after stopping the treatment.[8] Carry-over may be sought at the time of analysis and, if found, the study may be evaluated as a parallel group investigation using only data from the first phase. Recently concern has been expressed about the power of the tests to detect carry-over and the possible bias introduced by their use.[9] It is therefore important to design trials which will avoid carry-over as far as possible, generally by the inclusion of adequate washout phases between treatments.

Randomization and stratification are techniques to ensure that the different groups within a trial have a similar frequency of both known and unknown risk factors for the disease being studied. More sophisticated techniques have become available to enable a good balance to be achieved even with a small number of patients.[10] Even so, it is important that any imbalance between groups is looked for at the time of analysis.

The random-zero sphygmomanometer, which has been the tool for blood pressure measurement in most large trials, has come in for some recent criticism.[11] Unfortunately no other method of measuring blood pressure has been shown to be uniformly superior, and we believe that this will remain the practical gold standard for some time. The introduction of non-invasive automated measurement of blood pressure may give further insights into the diurnal variation of blood pressure and provide a large number of blood pressure readings, but the superiority of the presently available devices over standard measurement techniques is not established. Although the ambulatory devices have improved considerably, it is clear that they are inaccurate during exercise and probably only as accurate as the traditional random zero sphygmomanometer at rest. The frequency of blood pressure measurement in a long-term trial may alter the variance of the estimate of treatment effect. Multiple measurements of blood pressure at a single visit provide information about the accuracy of the measurement technique but little about the longer term variability of the blood pressure.[12] It is therefore better to have the blood pressure measured at a number of separate clinic visits. Thus, in a practical trial of six weeks treatment duration, it is better to have two visits during the run in phase (weeks -1 and 0) and two during the treatment phase (weeks 5 and 6) rather than increasing the number of blood pressure measurements at single visit.

New drug *versus* placebo

Power= 0.9
Significance = 0.05
Difference to be detected = 21/10mmHg = MAP 13.7
Expected S.D. of MAP = 9mmHg

Sample size required* = 20 (10 active, 10 placebo); (*add 20% for drop-outs).

Fig.2. Example (single B.P. measurements)

When designing a clinical trial one of the critical factors in the minds of the investigators is its size because they have the difficult task of recruiting all those patients. This depends not only on the magnitude of the effect sought, but also the desired power, significance level and the variance of the blood pressure measurement (approximately 9 mmHg for standard clinic random zero readings). Amongst these the power of the study is really of fundamental importance because this will determine the likelihood of the trial coming to the correct conclusion. Often trial size is determined by the practicalities of patient recruitment and the investigators are then disappointed when the outcome fails to demonstrate a definitive result. Several charts or algorithms[13,14] have been published to avoid any major mathematics in calculating trial sizes and an example of a typical calculation is given in figure 2. Recently emphasis on expressing results in terms of confidence intervals has led to a new method for calculating sample sizes which leads to smaller numbers of patients required.[15] This is not without its critics and we believe should not be widely adopted until the method has been more thoroughly investigated.

Finally a little needs to be said about the clinical significance of the results. With so much attention on the technical details of trial design and statistical analysis it is simple to overlook the ways in which the data will eventually be used. Poor trial design is capable of producing a result in which a clinically important result is overlooked, but the converse is also the case in that a large trial may demonstrate a result of high statistical significance when the magnitude of the treatment effect is so small as to make it clinically irrelevant. Thus in a placebo controlled trial of ketanserin[16] a significant effect of the drug on blood pressure was demonstrated, yet the size of the effect was so much smaller than that with atenolol or bendrofluazide as to make it clinically of little value.

References

1. European Working Party: Mortality and morbidity results from the European Working Party on High Blood Pressure in the Elderly Trial. Lancet 1985; 1:1349

96

2. The Management Committee: The Australian therapeutic trial in mild hypertension. Lancet 1980; 1:1261

3. Medical Research Council Working Party: MRC trial of treatment of mild hypertension: principal results. Br. Med. J. 1985; 191:97

4. Veterans Administration Cooperative Study Group: Effects of treatment on morbidity in hypertension II. Results in patients with diastolic blood pressure averaging 90 through 114mmHg. JAMA 1970; 213:1143

5. Collins R., Peto R., MacMahon S. et al.: Blood pressure, stroke, and coronary heart disease. 2: Short-term reductions in blood pressure: overview of randomised drug trials in their epidemiological context. Lancet 1990;335:827

6. Intersalt Cooperative Research Group: Intersalt: an international study of electrolyte excretion and blood pressure. Results for 24hr urinary sodium and potassium excretion. Br. Med. J. 1988; 297: 319

7. Watt G.C.M., Edwards C., Hart J.T., Hart M., Walton P., Foy C.J.W.: Dietary sodium restriction for mild hypertension in general practice. Br. Med. J. 1983; 286: 432

8. Endres S., Ghorboni R., Kelley V.E. et al.: The effect of dietary supplementation with n-3 polyunsaturated fatty acids on the synthesis of interleukin I and tumor necrosis factor by mononuclear cells. New Engl. J. Med. 1989; 320 (5): 265-271

9. Armitage P.: Should we cross off the crossover? Br. J. Clin. Pharmac. 1991; 32:1

10. Chaput de Saintonge D.M., Evans S.J.W., Vere D.W.: Statistical methods in clinical trials. In *Recent Advances in Clinical Pharmacology,* London, Edinburgh, Churchill Livingstone 1990; 19-34

11. O'Brien E., Mee F., Atkins F., O'Malley K.: Inaccuracy of the Hawksley random zero sphygmomanometer. Lancet 1990; 2:1465

12. Armitage P., Rose G.A.: The variability of measurements of casual blood pressure. Clin. Sci. 1966; 30:325

13. Altman D.G.: Statistics and ethics in medical research. III. How large a sample? Br. Med. J. 1980; 281: 1336

14. Freestone S., Silas J.H., Ramsay L.E.: Sample size for short-term trials of antihypertensive drugs. Br. J. Clin. Pharmac. 1982; 14:265

15. Bristol D.R.: Sample sizes for constructing confidence intervals and testing hypotheses. Statistics in Medicine. 1989; 8:803

16. Cameron H.A., Waller P.C., Ramsay L.E.: Ketanserin in essential hypertension: use as monotherapy and in combination with a diuretic or β-adrenoceptor antagonist. Br. J. Clin. Pharmac. 1987; 24:705

15. Eicosanoid Dependent and Independent Effects of n-3 Fatty Acids on Platelets and Vascular Function

G.A. FitzGerald

Center for Cardiovascular Science, Department of Medicine and Experimental Therapeutics, University College Dublin, Mater Hospital, Dublin, Ireland

Introduction

Fish oils have been recognized as potentially important modulators of platelet function and vascular tone. Initially, their influence on eicosanoid synthesis was believed to be responsible for most, if not all, of their physiological effects. However, more recent evidence has challenged this view and the principal data on this subject will be reviewed.

Fish Oils, Platelets and Vascular Function

Several studies indicate that fish oils cause a marked, but incomplete, depression of thromboxane (Tx) biosynthesis. This effect may be sufficient to explain the modest inhibitory effect of fish oils on platelet aggregation ex *vivo*,[1] as there is a nonlinear relationship between inhibition of platelet Tx formation and inhibition of Tx dependent platelet function.[2]

The administration of n-3 polyunsaturated fatty acids (PUFA) results in an increase of the ratio between eicosapentaenoic acid (EPA: n-3 20:5) and arachidonic acid (AA: n-6 20:4) in cell membranes; for example, this has been documented in animal studies in both platelets and in the vasculature.[3] In the same experiment, the reduction of basal Tx biosynthesis was incomplete despite high dose fish oil administration (Fig. 1). In this canine model, in which an experimentally induced coronary thrombus is lysed with recombinant tissue plasminogen activator (rt-PA)[3], chronic pretreatment with n-3 PUFA had a modest, but significant acceler-

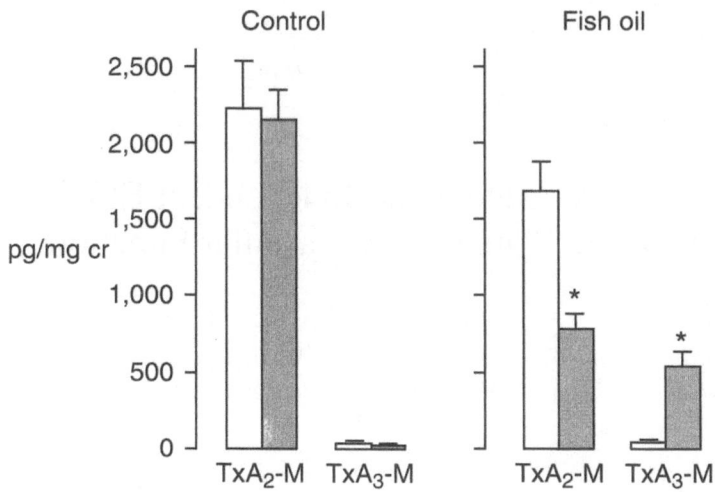

Fig. 1. Bar graph of basal production of thromboxanes A_2 and A_3 in groups of dogs fed standard lab chow (controls) or a low fat chow supplemented with fish oil corresponding to roughly 10 g EPA and 6.7 g DHA per day. Effects on thromboxanes are assessed by production of the 2,3-dinor-TxB$_2$ (TxA$_2$-M) and 2,3-dinor-17-ene-TxB$_2$ (TxA$_3$-M) metabolites in urine. Values are mean ± SEM in picograms/milligram creatinine. Open bars, baseline values; solid bars, values after 4 weeks of control or fish oil diet (*p<0.001).

ating effect on the time to reperfusion.[4] No effect on the incidence of re-occlusion was detected. However, it is interesting to note that in dogs pretreated with n-3 PUFA, the plasma concentration of tissue plasminogen activator measured during rt-PA infusion was increased compared to controls.

In patients with peripheral vascular disease, Tx formation is considerably elevated compared to healthy controls.[5] In these patients, supplementation with n-3 PUFA reduced Tx synthesis, but Tx formation remained elevated compared to untreated, healthy controls.[6]

The incomplete inhibition by n-3 PUFA supplementation of Tx synthesis is also evident in a study in patients undergoing percutaneous transluminal coronary angioplasty (Fig. 2).[7] In these patients, pretreatment with aspirin at two different dosages, 75 mg/day and 325 mg/day for at least 3 days, was able largely to suppress the increment in Tx synthesis associated with the procedure. Pretreatment for 3 weeks with high dose n-3 PUFA (10 g/day eicosapentaenoic acid), by contrast, only caused a moderate suppression of Tx synthesis.

However, several different pathways lead to platelet activation and it is possible that n-3 PUFA may also have an inhibitory effect on platelets that is independent of Tx formation. Recent studies have shown that n-3 PUFA supplementation inhibits the

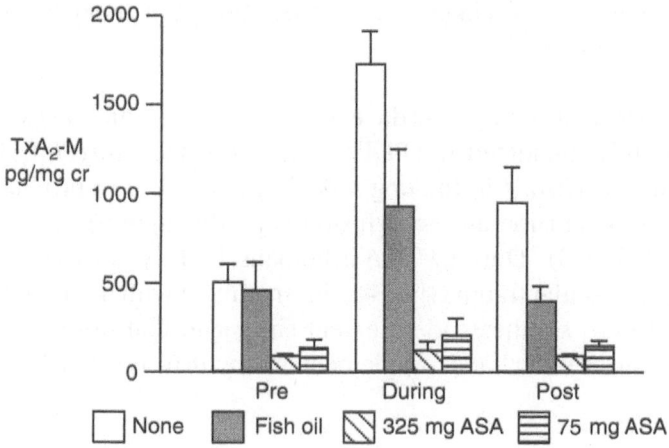

Fig. 2. Bar graph showing excretion of 2,3-dinor-thromboxane (Tx)B$_2$ (TxA$_2$-M) in successive 6-hour urinary aliquots commencing 6 hours before percutaneous transluminal coronary angioplasty. TxA$_2$-M excretion increased significantly in aspirin-sensitive patients (open bars; p<0.01) and in those pretreated with fish oil (p<0.05). Pretreatment with aspirin for 3 days on both regimens (325 mg and 75 mg per day), but not fish oil regimen, prevented the increase in TxA$_2$-M during angioplasty.

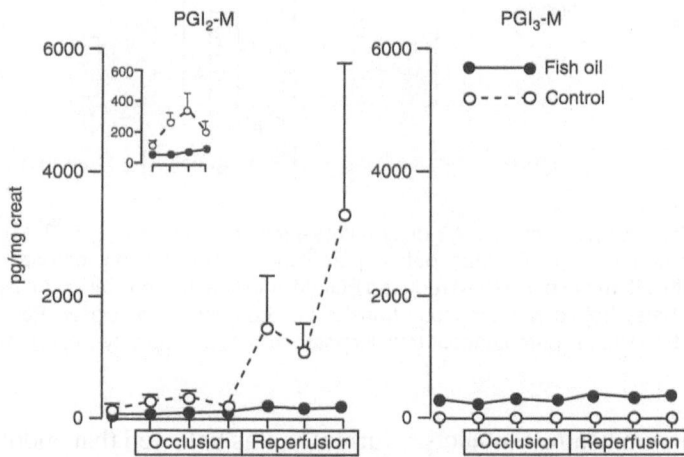

Fig. 3. Plots of stimulated production of prostaglandin (PG)I$_2$ and PGI$_3$ during coronary occlusion and reperfusion. Biosynthesis of these eicosanoids was assessed by production of 2,3-dinor-6-keto-PGF$_{1\alpha}$ (PGI$_2$-M) and 2,3-dinor-6-keto-17-ene-PGF$_{1\alpha}$ (PGI$_3$-M) metabolites in urine and expressed as picograms/milligram creatinine. Data are mean ± SEM. Insert: Expanded scale of prethrombosis and occlusion values of PGI$_2$-M. Time is expressed on the horizontal axis; each mark on this axis denotes 1 hour. There is no statistical change in PGI$_2$ or PGI$_3$ production with occlusion or reperfusion in the fish oil groups. There is an increase in PGI$_2$ production in controls for both of the events (p<0.02). Note the difference in scales for the PGI$_2$ and PGI$_3$ metabolites.

adhesion of platelets to collagen and exerts fibrinogen independent effects on platelet aggregation.[8]

Multiple mechanisms may transduce the effects of fish oil on vascular function and are not entirely elucidated. n-3 PUFA depress prostacyclin (PGI_2) formation by vascular tissues *in vitro*.[10] In the dog model, the increase in production of PGI_2 during coronary occlusion and reperfusion is partly suppressed by pretreatment with n-3 PUFA (Fig. 3).[7] During PTCA in humans, PGI_2 synthesis is also increased, probably due to vascular trauma (Fig. 4).[7] Pretreatment with n-3 PUFA inhibits this stimulation of PGI_2 synthesis to an extent similar to that observed with aspirin pretreatment. On the other hand, supplementation with n-3 PUFA does not suppress

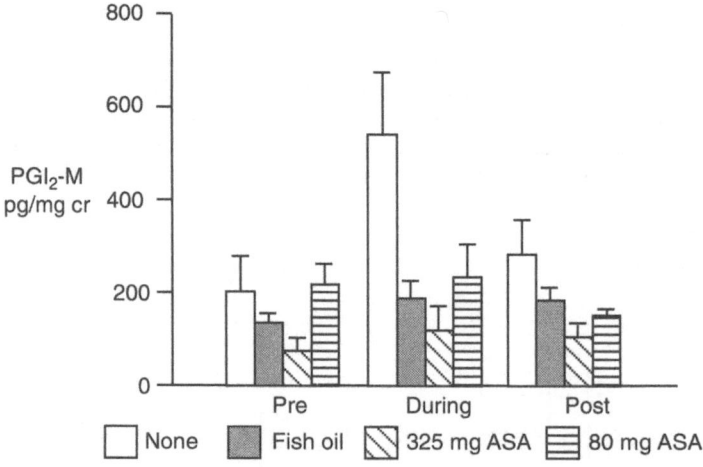

Fig. 4. Bar graph showing excretion of 2,3-dinor-6-keto -prostaglandin $(PG)F_{1\alpha}$ (PGI_2-M) in successive 6-hour aliquots commencing 6 hours before percutaneous transluminal coronary angioplasty. Pretreatment with 325 mg aspirin (ASA) reduced PGI_2-M significantly from values in aspirin-sensitive controls (open bars) before percutaneous transluminal coronary angioplasty. PGI_2-M increased significantly ($p<0.01$) during percutaneous transluminal coronary angioplasty only in the control group.

PGI_2 formation in healthy subjects.[6] Currently, it is believed that endothelial PGI_2 formation is a reactive, possibly homeostatic, process. Detection of a suppression of stimulated, but not basal, PGI_2 formation by fish oil may be analogous to suppression of stimulated endothelial PGI_2 formation by endothelial cells *in vitro* by n-3 fatty acids. The relationship of these observations to the direct inhibitory effects of fish oil on vascular reactivity,[11] proliferative occlusion of vascular grafts[12] or dietary induction of atherosclerosis in several species[13,14] remains to be established.

It is interesting to note that in a recent study in which supplementation with n-3 PUFA to patients with mild hypertension caused a modest, but significant reduction of diastolic blood pressure, alterations in PGI_2 or PGE_2 formation did not correlate with the changes in blood pressure.[15] Thus, there is no clearcut relation between the antihypertensive effect of n-3 PUFA and their effect on biosynthesis of these vasodilator eicosanoids. n-3 PUFA may modify vascular function by mechanisms independent of eicosanoids. For example, endothelium relaxant activity is reportedly enhanced by n-3 supplementation[16] and expression of growth factor-like activity is modulated.[17] This may relate not only to the inhibition of vascular proliferation in several species,[13,14,18,19] but also to an apparent antiangiogenic effect of fish oils.[20] An inhibitory effect on thromboxane receptor expression has been documented in vitro,[21,22] but has not been replicated *ex vivo* in man (Clarke R.J. and FitzGerald G.A.; unpublished data).

Finally, a potentially important mechanism by which eicosanoids may be relevant to the effects of n-3 PUFA on platelets and blood vessels may be via the P450 dependent metabolism of arachidonic acid. This pathway leads to formation of epoxyeicosatrienoic acid (EET) derivatives that have been shown to be important in mediating mitogenic responses.[23,24] Recently, we have observed that EET biosynthesis is increased during coronary angioplasty in humans and that this increase is significantly prevented by fish oil treatment.[25] These observations open new perspectives for a thorough understanding of the eicosanoid dependent effects of n-3 PUFA on platelets and vascular function.

References

1. FitzGerald G.A., Price P., Knapp H.R.: Biochemical and functional effects of dietary substrate modification in man. In: Simopoulos A., Kifer D. (Eds.) *Health Effects of Polyunsaturated Fatty Acids in Seafoods.* New York, Academic Press. 1986; 61-77
2. Reilly I.A.G., FitzGerald G.A.: Inhibition of thromboxane formation *in vivo* and *ex vivo*: implications for therapy with platelet inhibitory drugs. Blood 1987; 69: 180-186
3. FitzGerald D.J., Wright F., FitzGerald G.A.: Increased thromboxane biosynthesis during coronary thrombolysis: Evidence that thromboxane A_2 modulates the response to tissue-type plasminogen activator *in vivo*. Circ. Res. 1989; 65:83-94
4. Braden G., Knapp H.R., FitzGerald D.J., FitzGerald, G.A.: Dietary fish oil accelerates the response to coronary thrombolysis with tissue-plasminogen activator: evidence for an antithrombotic effect *in vivo*. Circulation 1990; 82: 178-187
5. Reilly I.A.G., Doran J., Smith B., FitzGerald G.A.: Increased thromboxane biosynthesis in a human model of platelet activation: biochemical and functional consequences of selective inhibition of thromboxane synthase. Circulation 1986; 73: 1300-1309
6. Knapp H.R., Reilly I.A.G., Alessandrini P., FitzGerald G.A.: *In vivo* indexes of platelet and vascular function during fish-oil administration in patients with atherosclerosis. N. Engl. J. Med. 1986; 314: 937-943

7. Braden G., Knapp H.R. FitzGerald G.A.: Suppression of eicosanoid formation during coronary angioplasty by fish oil and aspirin. Circulation 1991; 84: 679-685

8. Xiaolin L. and Steiner M.: Fish Oil: A potent inhibitor of platelet adhesiveness. Blood 1990; 76: 938-945

9. Xiaolin L., Steiner M.: Dose response of dietary fish oil supplementations on platelet adhesion. Arteriosclerosis Thromb. 1991; 11: 39-46

10. Yerram N.R., Spector A.A.: Effects of omega-3 fatty acids on vascular smooth muscle cells: reduction in arachidonic acid incorporation into inositol phospholipids. Lipids 1989; 24: 594-602

11. Malis C.D., Leaf A., Varadarajan G.S., Newell J.B., Weber P.C., Force T., Bonventre J.V.: Effects of dietary 2,3 fatty acids on vascular contractility in preanoxic and postanoxic aortic rings. Circulation 1991; 84: 1393-1401

12. Sarris G.E., Fann J.l., Sokoloff M.H., Smith D.L., Loveday M., Kosek J.C., Stephens R.J., Cooper A.D., May K., Willis A.L., Miller D.C.: Mechanisms responsible for inhibition of vein-graft arteriosclerosis by fish oil. Circulation 1989; 80:1109-1123

13. Davis H.R., Bridenstine R.T., Vesselinovitch D., Wissler R.W.: Fish oil inhibits development of atherosclerosis in rhesus monkeys. Arteriosclerosis 1987; 7: 441-449

14. Zhu B-Q., Sievers R.E., Isenberg W.M., Smith D.L., Parmley W.W.: Regression of atherosclerosis in cholesterol-fed rabbits: effects of fish oil and verapamil. J. Am. Coll. Cardiol. 1990; 15: 231-237

15. Knapp H.R., FitzGerald G.A.: The antihypertensive effects of fish oil: a controlled study of polyunsaturated fatty acid supplements in essential hypertension. N. Engl. J. Med. 1989; 320:1037-1043

16. Shimokawa H., Vanhoutte P.M.: Dietary n-3 fatty acids and endothelium dependent relaxations in porcine coronary arteries. Am. J. Physiol. 1989; 256: H968-H973

17. Fox P.L., DiCorleto P.D.: Fish oils inhibit endothelial cell production of platelet-derived growth factor-like protein. Science 1988; 241: 453-456

18. Sassen L.M.A., Konig M.M.G., Dekkers D.H.W., Lamers J.M.J., Verdouw P.D.: Differential effects of n-3 fatty acids on the regression of atherosclerosis in coronary arteries and the aorta of the pig. Eur. Heart J. 1989; 10: 173-178

19. Sarris G.E., Mitchell R.S., Billingham M.E., Glasson J.R., Cahill P.D., Miller D.C.: Inhibition of accelerated cardiac allograft arteriosclerosis by fish oil. J. Thorac. Cardiovasc. Surg. 1989; 97: 841-855

20. Kanayasu T., Morita I., Nakao-Hayashi J., Asuwa N., Fujisawa C., Ishil T., Ito H., Murota S.I.: Eicosapentaenoic acid inhibits tube formation of vascular endothelial cells in vitro. Lipids 1991; 26: 271-276

21. Swann P.G., Venton D.L., Le Breton G.C.: Eicosapentaenoic acid and docosahexaenoic acid are antagonists at the thromboxane A_2/prostaglandin H_2 receptor in human platelets. FEBS Letters 1989; 243: 244-246

22. Swann P.G., Parent C.A., Croset M., Fonlupt P., Lagarde M., Venton D.L., LeBreton G.C.: Enrichment of platelet phospholipids with eicosapentaenoic acid and docosahexaenoic acid inhibits thromboxane A_2/prostaglandin H_2 receptor binding and function. J. Biol. Chem. 1990; 265: 21692-21697

23. Sellmayer A., Uedelhoven W.M., Weber P.C., Bonventre J.V.: Endogenous noncyclooxygenase metabolites of arachidonic acid modulate growth and mRNA levels of immediate-early response genes in rat mesangial cells. J. Biol. Chem. 1991; 266: 3800-3807

24. Force T., Hyman G., Hajjar R., Sellmayer A., Bonventre J.V. Noncyclooxygenase metabolites of arachidonic acid amplify the vasopressin induced Ca^{2+} signal in glomerular mesangial cells by releasing Ca^{2+} from intracellular stores. J. Biol. Chem. 1991; 266: 4295-4302

25. Braden G.R., FitzGerald G.A.: Coronary angioplasty stimulates biosynthesis of cytochrome P450 monoxygenase products in humans. Clin. Res. 1991; 39:183A

16. n-3 Fatty Acids in Hypertension

K. H. Bønaa

Institute of Community Medicine, University of Tromsø, Breivika, Norway

Supported by the Norwegian Council on Cardiovascular Diseases, the Norwegian Fishermen Sales Organization, and Norsk Hydro.

Clustering of Coronary Heart Disease Risk Factors in Hypertension

Hypertensive subjects are at increased risk for coronary heart disease (CHD). Although this may be due to the consequences of an elevated blood pressure per se, it is well known that hypertension frequently is associated with other CHD risk factors that may contribute as well. Kjeldsen et al. observed that blood platelets from subjects with high blood pressure possessed hypersensitivity to adrenaline, and suggested that enhanced platelet activation in essential hypertension was related to raised sympathetic adrenergic tone.[1]

The Tromsø Study further shows that there is a linear association between the level of blood pressure and serum cholesterol (Fig. 1) and triglyceride concentrations throughout the usual range of blood pressure in a population.[2] These relationships were found to be independent of potential confounding factors such as sex, age, body weight, physical activity, or alcohol consumption. Increased sympathetic drive and/or insulin resistance may partly account for the relationships between blood pressure and serum lipids,[3,4] but it is also possible that hyperlipidemia per se contribute to high blood pressure by modulating endothelial cell functioning.[5]

There is increasing evidence of a role for triglyceride-rich lipoproteins in atherogenesis. Hypertriglyceridemia has also been associated with high levels of activated Factor VII phospholipid complexes (PLC-factor VII).[6] This activity has been correlated with the risk of cardiovascular disease.[6]

The clustering of cardiovascular risk factors in hypertension may partly account for the failure of CHD mortality to respond to blood pressure reduction, and it suggests that single risk factor intervention may be inadequate to prevent CHD in

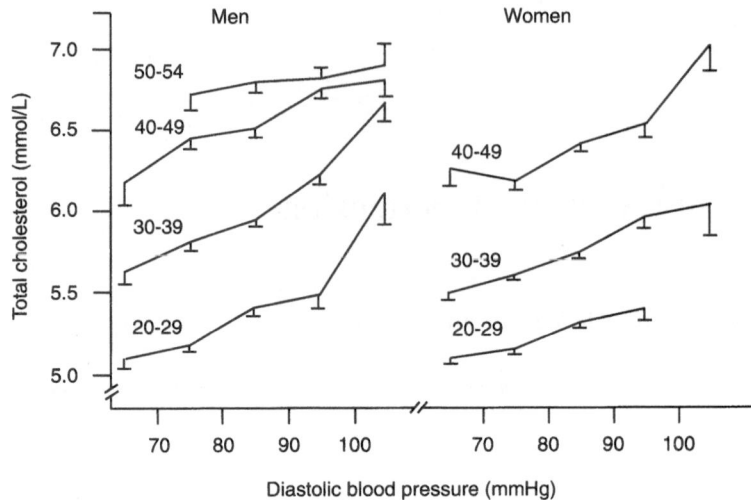

Fig. 1. The Tromsø study; plot of mean concentrations of serum total cholesterol levels *vs* diastolic blood pressure in men 20-29, 30-39, 40-49, and 50-54 years old and in women 20-29, 30-39, and 40-49 years old. Cells with less than 20 observations were pooled with adjacent category. T bars are SEM.

hypertension. n-3 polyunsaturated fatty acids (PUFA) have been reported to exert favorable effects on platelets, blood lipids, and a variety of biochemical factors that may be associated with cardiovascular disease.[7] These effects may be of particular value in a multifactorial disorder such as hypertension.

n-3 Fatty Acids in Hypertension

In 1985 the first report appeared indicating that adding fatty fish to the diet of patients with mild hypertension lowered their blood pressure.[8] However, decades of experience in the design of drug trials for antihypertensive agents have left few marks in the field of n-3 PUFA and blood pressure. In a search of peer-reviewed English journals in the period from 1970 to 1988 Radack and Deck found 22 studies reporting blood-pressure effects of n-3 fatty acids,[8] but they nevertheless concluded that "little scientifically valid evidence is available to demonstrate a significant blood pressure-lowering effect of n-3 fatty acids". The Authors noted that only one[9] randomized, controlled investigation studied hypertensive subjects. During the last two years, however, four randomized studies have suggested a modest antihypertensive effect of n-3 fatty acids in human hypertension,[10-13] while one study was inconclusive.[14]

Table I summarizes randomized, controlled studies with fish oil in human hypertension. The overall result indicates that 3.6 g/day of eicosapentaenoic acid (EPA; 20:5n-3) and 2.1 g/day of docosahexaenoic acid (DHA; 22:6n-3) lower

:105

Table I. Dose of n-3 fatty acids and individual effect sizes in six randomized studies with fish oil in human hypertension.

Study (ref)	Group[a]	n	Total	EPA	DHA	Pre	Change	Pre	Change
			Dose of oil (g/day)			Systolic BP (mmHg)		Diastolic BP (mmHg)	
Norris[9]	Fish oil	8	16.5	3.0	2.0	160.0	-9.0	94.0	-1.5
	Control	8	16.5			160.0	+1.0	94.0	+0.5
Knapp[10]	Fish oil	8	50.0	9.0	6.0	138.7	-6.5	94.3	-4.4
	Fish oil	8	10.0	1.8	1.2	137.0	-0.9	94.6	-0.4
	Control[b]	16	50.0			135.2	+2.0	93.4	+0.9
Bønaa[11]	Fish oil	79	6.0	3.3	1.8	144.9	-4.6	95.0	-3.0
	Control	78	6.0			142.8	+1.2	94.6	-0.2
Levinson[12]	Fish oil	8	50.0	9.0	6.0	149.0	-8.0	91.0	-10.0
	Control	8	50.0			147.0	-3.0	90.0	+1.0
Radack[13]	Fish oil	16	6.0	1.2	0.8	136.9	-6.5	96.4	-4.4
	Control	17	6.0			135.6	+0.7	93.4	+2.3
Meland[14]	Fish oil	20	20.0	3.6	2.4	147.0	-4.0	101.0	-4.0
	Control	20	20.0			150.0	-5.0	101.0	-3.0
Weighted[c] Means	Fish oil	146		3.6	2.1	144.6	-5.1	95.6	-3.5
	95% CI						-7.3,-2.9		-4.3,-2.7
	Control	147				142.2	+0.1	94.9	-0.1
	95% CI						-2.1,+2.3		-0.9,+0.7

a: Control groups received placebo (constituents not given),[9] safflower oil,[10,13] corn oil,[11] or a mixture of oils.[10,12,14]
b: The study included two control groups. The pooled results are shown.
c: Dose of n-3 fatty acids and blood presssure were weighted by the number of participants in each study to give an overall per subject (not per study) mean. 95%CI were estimated from the pooled SD (13.5 and 5.1 mmHg for systolic and diastolic BP, respectively).
EPA, eicosapentaenoic (20:5n-3) acid; DHA, docosahexaenoic (22:6n-3) acid; BP, blood pressure; CI, confidence interval.

systolic blood pressure by 5.1 mmHg (95% confidence interval -7.3, -2.9) and diastolic blood pressure by 3.5 mmHg (95% confidence interval -4.3, -2.7) in mild hypertension.

The Tromsø Study

We conducted a population-based, randomized, 10-week dietary-supplementation trial in which the effects of 6 g per day of fish oil supplied as ethylesters were compared with those of 6 g per day of corn oil in 157 men and women with previously untreated stable, mild essential hypertension (Fig. 2).[11] The primary end-point was a change in blood pressure. We also examined the effects on serum lipids and the phospholipase C-sensitive fraction of Factor VII activity (PLC-factor VII). PLC-factor VII activity was evaluated with a Normotest assay after exposure of plasma to phospholipase C as described by Dalaker et al.[15] We monitored diet and assessed concentrations of plasma phospholipid fatty acids to determine the relation between diet, fatty acids, and blood pressure.

The mean systolic blood pressure fell by 4.6 mmHg (95% confidence interval -7.4, -1.8; p=0.002), and diastolic pressure by 3.0 mmHg (95% confidence interval -4.5, -1.5; p=0.0002) in the group receiving n-3 PUFA; there was no significant change in the group receiving corn oil. The differences between the groups remained significant for both systolic (6.4 mmHg; p=0.0025) and diastolic (2.8

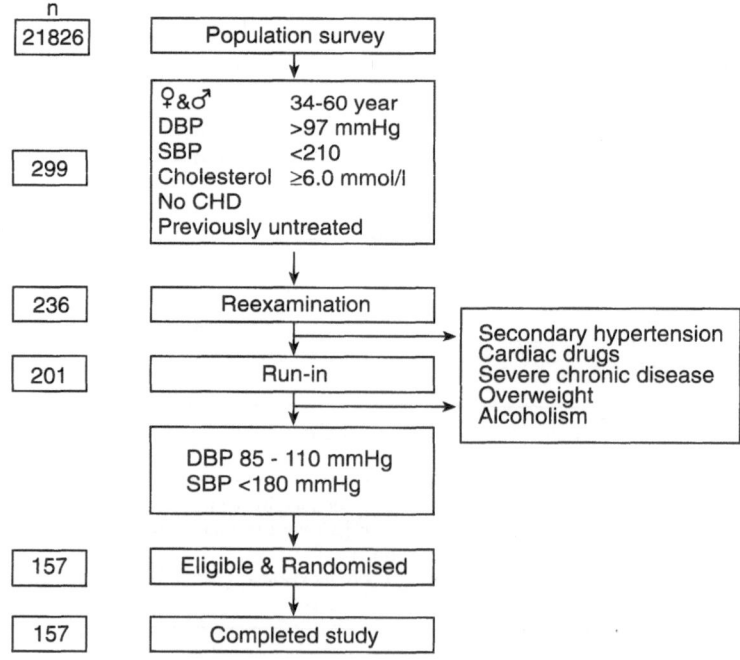

Fig. 2. The Tromsø study; chart showing number of participants and eligibility criteria for a population-based intervention trial with fish oil.[11]

mmHg; p=0.029) pressure after control for anthropometric, lifestyle, and dietary variables.

Base-line blood pressure was lower among those that consumed three or more fish dishes per week in their usual diet as compared to those that consumed less fish.[11] Subjects who consumed low amounts of fish in their usual diet had a greater rise in plasma phospholipid n-3 fatty acids and a greater fall in blood pressure than those who consumed more fish. The fall in blood pressure was larger as concentrations of plasma phospholipid n-3 fatty acids increased (Fig. 3).

The overall compliance with the study protocol was satisfactory, although 10 and 7 subjects respectively in the fish oil and corn oil groups reported that they did not take the prescribed number of capsules. Among subjects consuming less than three fish dishes per week in their habitual diet who took the prescribed dose of fish oil (n=35) systolic and diastolic pressures fell by 8.7 and 4.2 mmHg, respectively. In contrast, systolic and diastolic blood pressure increased by 4.4 and 2.1 mmHg among subjects consuming less than three fish dishes per week who took the prescribed dose of corn oil (n=32).

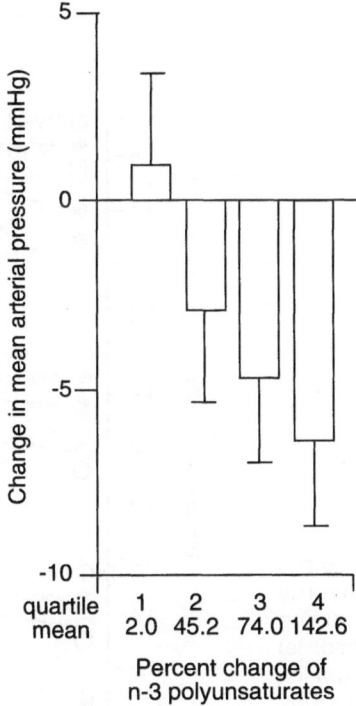

Fig. 3. The Tromsø study; changes in mean arterial pressure during 10 weeks dietary supplementation with fish oil according to changes in plasma phospholipid n-3 fatty acid concentrations. Each bar represents the mean (SEM) value of 19 observations (adjusted for age, sex, smoking, and change in body weight during the study).

Serum triglycerides fell by 20.3 percent from 1.48 to 1.18 mmol/l in the fish oil group. n-3 PUFA lowered triglycerides in men and women, smokers and non-smokers, and in persons with low or high levels of EPA at base-line (Fig. 4).

Men had higher PLC-factor VII activity than women before supplementation. The mean PLC-factor VII activity decreased from 8.2% to 4.9% (p<0.05) in men who received fish oil, whereas it did not change in women (4.5 percent at base-line vs 5.4 percent after 10 weeks) or in those who received corn oil. There was a significant correlation (r=0.45; p=0.003) between the fall in serum triglyceride concentration and the decline in PLC-factor VII activity among men taking fish oil.

Comments

The Tromsø study shows that n-3 fatty acids may have beneficial effects on several risk factors associated with atherosclerosis and coagulation. The blood pressure-lowering effect in the total study group was modest, but subjects who had a larger rise in level of plasma phospholipid n-3 PUFA showed a fall in blood pressure that may be of clinical significance. The lower blood pressure at base-line

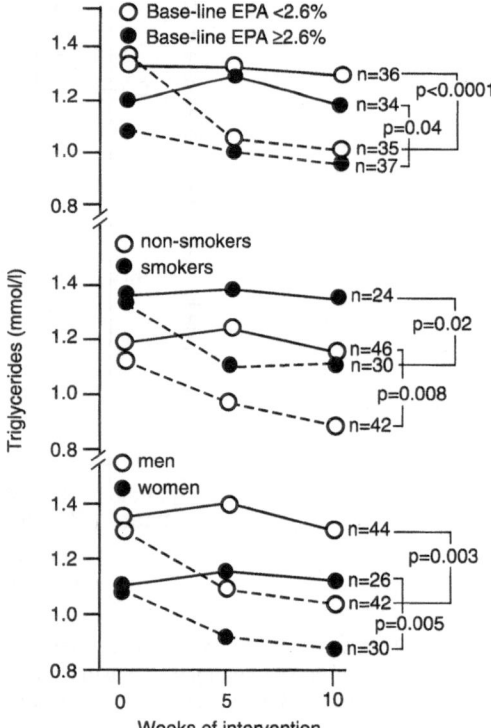

Fig. 4 The Tromsø study; line graphs showing adjusted geometric mean values for serum triglycerides (TG) during supplementation with fish oil (dashed line) or corn oil (solid line) in subgroups divided according to the median base-line level of plasma phospholipid eicosapentaenoic acid (EPA) (adjusted for gender and smoking), smoking status (adjusted for gender and EPA), or gender (adjusted for EPA and smoking).

in subjects who habitually consumed larger quantities of fish further suggests that dietary enrichment with n-3 PUFA would be important from the primary prevention standpoint. Although this finding also may indicate that the effects of n-3 PUFA on blood pressure is sustained over time, this hypothesis was not tested adequately in the intervention trials (Table I) which only lasted for 4 to 12 weeks.

The data presented in Table I provide strong evidence that the blood pressure-lowering effect of polyunsaturated fat is restricted to the n-3 family. Fish oil may be less effective than antihypertensive drugs in lowering the blood pressure. We do not know, however, to what level blood pressure should be lowered in mild or moderate hypertension to optimize treatment. Table I indicates that diastolic blood pressure is reduced by 2.7 to 4.3 mmHg after fish oil. In comparison, the diastolic blood pressure reduction was 5 to 6 mmHg in 14 unconfounded randomized trials with antihypertensive drugs.[16]

In prospective observational studies, a long-term difference of 5-6 mmHg in usual diastolic blood pressure is associated with about 35-40% less stroke and 20-25% less CHD.[16] However, whereas antihypertensive drug treatment reduced stroke incidence by 42%, the reduction in CHD was only 14%.[16] Whether fish oil alone or in combination with antihypertensive drugs may give a better result can only be tested in a large-scale prospective study. Such a study should probably include subjects with a combination of cardiovascular risk factors because they may be particularly likely to benefit from the multiple effects of fish oil.

There is evidence that the effect of fish oil on blood pressure is mediated by eicosapentaenoic and/or docosahexaenoic acid.[11] We do not know, however, if the two fatty acids are equally important and whether their effects on blood pressure are through the same mechanisms. It is possible that n-3 PUFA lower blood pressure by shifting the balance between vasoconstrictive and vasodilatory eicosanoids and/or by modulating the physicochemical properties of cell membranes so that signal transduction is altered. The relationship between n-3 PUFA and blood pressure is likely to be complex, and it is possible that hypertensives may respond differently to fish oil depending on other dietary as well as nondietary factors.

More work is needed to define the optimal dose of n-3 PUFA that lowers blood pressure with a minimum of side effects. Subjects with hypertension received on average 5.7 g PUFA per day during the trials (Table I). This dose is 30-fold greater than the amount of n-3 PUFA consumed by North american men in their usual diet.[17] Long term consumption of large amounts of the highly unsaturated n-3 PUFA may increase the formation of reactive oxygen species which may damage cellular membranes and increase the susceptibility of low density lipoprotein to oxidative changes.[7] Although these potential adverse effects may be prevented by increasing the dietary intake of antioxidants such as vitamin E, the longterm consequences of increased antioxidant requirements remain unknown.

The blood pressure lowering effect of n-3 PUFA now represents a relatively well-

110

documented effect of fish oil on a known risk factor for cardiovascular disease. Further studies are needed to find out if there is a place for n-3 PUFA in the prevention or treatment of hypertension.

References

1. Kjeldsen S.E., Gjesdal K., Eide I., Aakeson I., Amundsen R., Foss O.P., Leren P.: Increased beta-thromboglobulin in essential hypertension: interactions between arterial plasma adrenaline, platelet function and blood lipids. Acta Med. Scand. 1983; 213:369-373
2. Bønaa K.H., Thelle D.: Association between blood pressure and serum lipids in a population. The Tromsø Study. Circulation 1991;83:1305-1314.
3. Bravo E.L.: Metabolic factors and the sympathetic nervous system. Am. J. Hypertens. 1989; 2:339S-344S
4. Reaven G.M., Hoffman B.B.: Hypertension as a disease of carbohydrate and lipoprotein metabolism. Am. J. Med. 1989; 87(suppl 6A):2S-6S
5. Lüscher T.F.: Functional abnormalities of the vascular endothelium in hypertension and athero-sclerosis. Scand. J. Clin. Lab. Invest. Suppl. 1990; 50:28-32
6. Mann K.G.: Factor VII assays, plasma triglyceride levels, and cardiovascular disease risk. Arteriosclerosis 1989; 9:783-4
7. Leaf A., Weber P.C.: Cardiovascular effects of n-3 fatty acids. N. Engl. J. Med. 1988; 318:549-57
8. Radack K., Deck C.: The effects of omega-3 polyunsaturated fatty acids on blood pressure: a methodologic analysis of the evidence. J. Am. Coll. Nutr. 1989; 8:376-85
9. Norris P.G., Jones C.H.J., Weston M.J.: Effect of dietary supplementation with fish oil on systolic blood pressure in hypertension. Br. Med. J. 1986; 293:104-5
10. Knapp H.R., FitzGerald G.A.: The antihypertensive effects of fish oil. A controlled study of poyunsaturated fatty acid supplementation in essential hypertension. N. Engl. J. Med. 1989; 320:1037-43
11. Bønaa K.H., Bjerve K.S., Straume B., Gram I.T., Thelle D.: Effect of eicosapentaenoic and docosahexaenoic acids on blood pressure in hypertension. A population-based intervention trial from the Tromsø Study. N. Engl. J. Med. 1990; 322:795-801
12. Levinson P.D., Iosiphidis A.H., Saritelli A.L., Herbert P.N., Steiner M.: Effects of n-3 fatty acids in hypertension. Am. J. Hypertens. 1990; 3:754-60
13. Radack K., Deck C., Husten G.: The effects of low doses of n-3 fatty acid supplementation on blood pressure in hypertensive subjects. A randomized controlled trial. Arch. Intern. Med. 1991; 151:1173-80
14. Meland E., Fugelli P., Lalrum E., Ronneberg R., Sandvik L.: Effect of fish oil on blood pressure and blood lipids in men with mild to moderate hypertension. Scand. J. Prim. Health Care 1989; 7:131-5
15. Dalaker K., Janson T.L., Johnsen B., Skartlien A.H., Prydz H.: A simple method for determination of the factor VII phospholipid complex using Normotest. Thromb. Res. 1987; 47:87-93
16. Collins R., Peto R., MacMahon S., Hebert P., Fiebach N.H., Eberlein K.A., Godwin J, Qizilbash N, Taylor JO, Hennekens CH.: Blood pressure, stroke, and coronary heart disease. Part 2, Short-term reductions in blood pressure: overview of randomized drug trials in their epidemiological context. Lancet 1990;335:827-38
17. Dolecek T.A., Grandits G.: Dietary polyunsaturated fatty acids and mortality in the Multiple Risk Factor Intervention Trial (MRFIT). In: Simopoulos A.P., Kifer R.R., Martin R.E., Barlow S.M. (Eds): *Health effects of omega-3 polyunsaturated fatty acids in seafoods.* World Rev. Nutr. Diet. Basel: Karger, 1991;66:205-16

17. n-3 Fatty Acids in Comparison and in Combination with Other Drugs in the Management of Mild Hypertension

P. SINGER
Stoffwechselklinik Lindenfels, Federal Republic of Germany

n-3 Fatty Acids and Blood Pressure

Several studies have evaluated the effect of n-3 fatty acids on blood pressure in normotensive subjects and in hypertensive patients. They have generally demonstrated a consistent decrease of blood pressure in hypertensive patients but less consistent results in normotensive persons.

Several mechanisms may be responsible for this effect. These include alterations in eicosanoid metabolism, a decrease in levels of intracellular calcium ions, an increase in intracellular levels of potassium, an increase in sodium excretion. Also a decrease in plasma norepinephrine concentration and a decrease of the vasoconstrictor response to norepinephrine may be of importance (Tab. I).

Surprisingly few data, however, have been collected on hemodynamic changes induced by n-3 fatty acids in hypertensive patients, and it is still unclear if a reduction in peripheral resistance occurs after intake of n-3 fatty acids.

n-3 Fatty Acids *Versus* Propranolol in the Treatment of Hypertension

There is a lack of data comparing in the same population the antihypertensive effect of n-3 fatty acids with that of other antihypertensive agents. It is also unclear whether the antihypertensive effect of n-3 fatty acids is additive to that of other antihypertensive treatments.

To answer this question, we recently completed a study in which patients with hypertension (Tab. II) were randomized to receive n-3 fatty acids (9 grams per day), propranolol (80 mg per day) or a combination of both (Tab. III).

Table I. Mechanisms of blood pressure-lowering effect by dietary n-3 fatty acids

Parameters	Effect	References
I. Eicosanoids		
Thromboxane A$_2$ *	-	(Singer,[1] Knapp[2])
Thromboxane A$_3$ *	+	(Knapp[2])
Prostaglandin I$_3$ *	+	(Knapp[2])
Prostaglandin I$_2$ *	(+)	(Knapp,[2] v. Schacky[3])
II. Catecholamines		
Plasma norepinephrine		
Normotensives	-	(Singer[4])
Hypertensives	-	(Urakaze[5])
Response to norepinephrine	-	(Lorenz[6])
Response to phenylephrine	-	(Knapp[7])
III. Electrolytes		
Intracellular calcium	-	(Locher[8], Haller[9])
Intracellular potassium	+	(Singer[4])
Sodium excretion	+	(Lorenz[6], Urakaze[5])
Serum sodium	-	(Singer[4])
Plasma renin activity		
Hypertensives	+	(Singer[4])
Eskimos	+	(Jørgensen[10])
IV. Hemodynamics		
Renal blood flow	+	(Düsing[13])
Baroreceptor reflex	(+)	(Düsing[13])
Microcirculation		
Blood viscosity	-	(Cartwright[11])
Erythrocyte flexibility	+	(Terano[12])

* measured as metabolite excretion or thromboxane or prostacyclin metabolites
+ or (+) = increased; - = decreased

In the first two groups, after the run-in period, treatment with each drug lasted 36 weeks, and afterwards the patients were switched to a placebo treatment. In the third group, propranolol was given during the first 12 weeks and then fish oil was added for another 12 weeks. The patients were then changed to propranolol + fish oil placebo and finally to a placebo preparation alone. This design allowed us to evaluate the antihypertensive efficacy of both drugs alone and in combination, and also to evaluate the reversibility of the changes observed.

113

Table II. Design of the present study.

Group P (n=16)
Run-in (4 weeks)
Propranolol, 80 mg/day (36 weeks)
Propranolol placebo (4 weeks)

Group F (n=15)
Run-in (4 weeks)
Fish oil, 9 g/day (36 weeks)
Fish oil placebo (4 weeks)

Group P + F (n=16)
Run-in (4 weeks)
Propranolol, 80 mg/day (12 weeks)
Propranolol, 80 mg/day + fish oil, 9 g/day (12 weeks)
Propranolol, 80 mg.day + fish oil placebo (12 weeks)
Propranolol placebo (4 weeks)

Table III. Characteristics of the patients in the three treatment groups.

47 male patients with mild essential hypertension

	n	Age (years)	Height (cm)	Weight (kg)
Group F (fish oil)	15	38.9±5.3	175±7	73.8±7.2
Group P (propranolol)	16	34.9±5.8	178±8	75.6±6.9
Group P+F (propranolol+fish oil)	16	35.6±6.1	176±9	74.3±7.5

Compliance to the treatment with fish oil (n-3 fatty acids) was confirmed by a significant increase in serum phospholipids of both eicosapentaenoic acid (EPA) and docosahexaenoic acid (DHA). Changes in blood pressure in the three groups are shown in figure 1. It is noteworthy that a significant and quite similar antihypertensive effect was observed with the two drugs. Furthermore, the combination of propranolol and n-3 fatty acids had the most pronounced effect on blood pressure. The decrease in blood pressure was reversible after stopping the treatments.

Determination of norepinephrine concentration in plasma demonstrated a significant reduction after treatment with both propranolol and n-3 fatty acids (Fig. 2). This decrease was higher when the drug combination was used. The two drugs, on the other hand, had opposite effects on renin activity which was increased by n-3 fatty

114

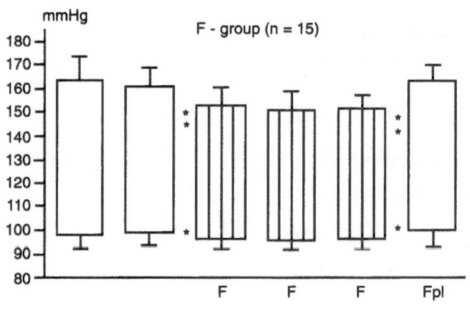

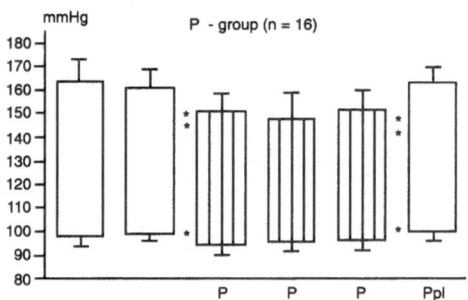

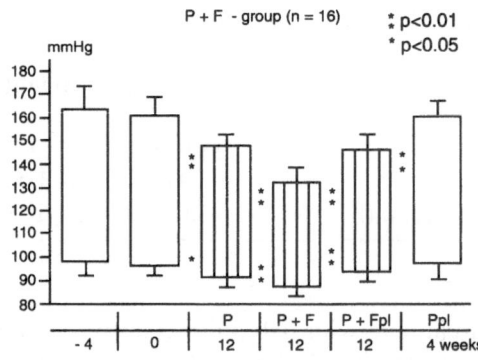

Fig. 1. Blood pressure (means with standard deviations) in patients with mild essential hypertension randomized to fish oil (group F), in patients randomized to treatment with propranolol (group P) and in patients given propranolol in combination with fish oil (group P + F), pl = placebo.

acids and decreased during propranolol treatment. The combination of the two drugs resulted in an increase in plasma renin activity. Thromboxane production was reduced by fish oil, in agreement with previous findings, and was also reduced by propranolol (Fig. 3). Again, the decrease in serum thromboxane formation after treatment with the combination of n-3 fatty acids and propranolol was greater than after either of the two treatments given separately.

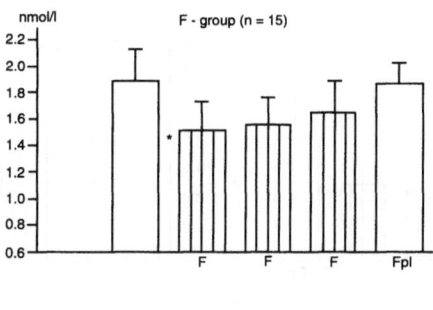

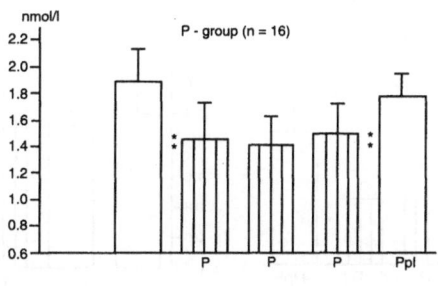

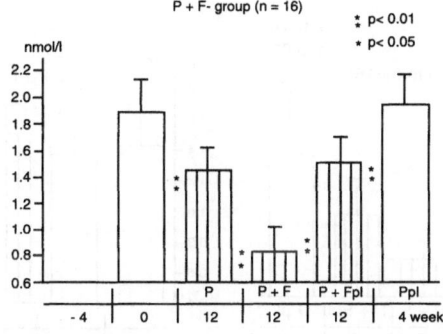

Fig. 2. Plasma norepinephrine in patients with mild essential hypertension randomized to fish oil (group F), propranolol (group P) and to propranolol in combination with fish oil (group P + F), pl = placebo.

Serum triglycerides significantly decreased after treatment with n-3 fatty acids contrasting a slight increase in triglycerides after propranolol. The drug combination resulted in a significant decrease of triglycerides in serum (Fig. 4). A reduction in total cholesterol and LDL-cholesterol was observed during fish oil treatment, and this was accompanied by a slight but significant increase in HDL-cholesterol (Fig. 5). The combination of drugs decreased total cholesterol and LDL-cholesterol, while HDL-cholesterol was increased.

116

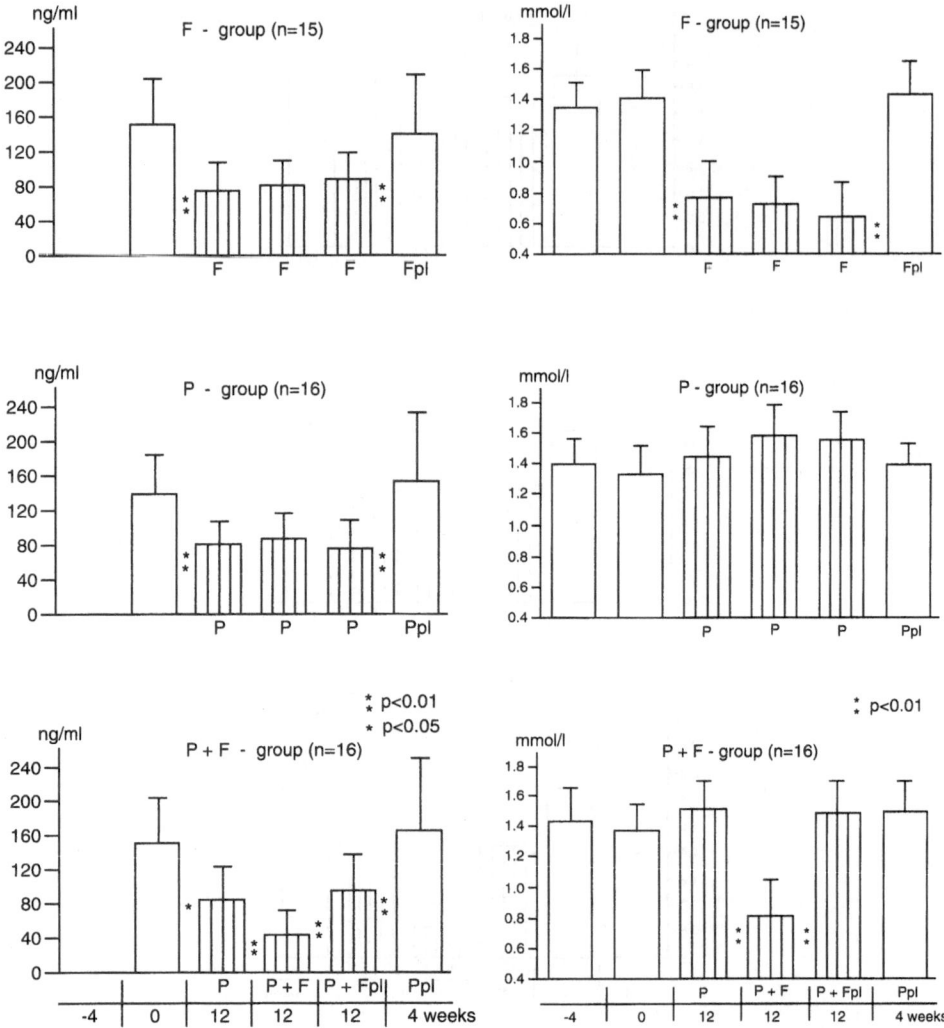

Fig. 3. Thromboxane formation in patients with mild essential hypertension randomized to fish oil (group F), propranolol (group P) and to propranolol in combination with fish oil (group P + F), pl=placebo.

Fig. 4. Serum triglycerides in patients with mild essential hypertension randomized to fish oil (group F), propranolol (group P) and to propranolol in combination with fish oil (group P + F), pl=placebo.

Conclusion of the Study

These results indicate that supplementation with n-3 fatty acids is an effective antihypertensive treatment. The decrease in blood pressure is comparable to that obtained with propranolol at least with the doses studied. Furthermore, the antihypertensive effect of n-3 fatty acids is accompanied by an effect on the lipid

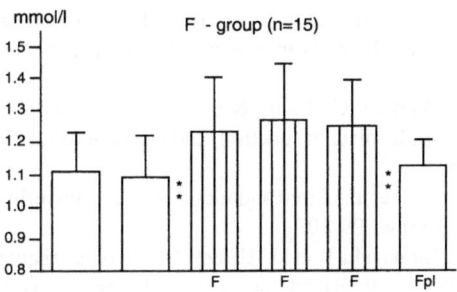

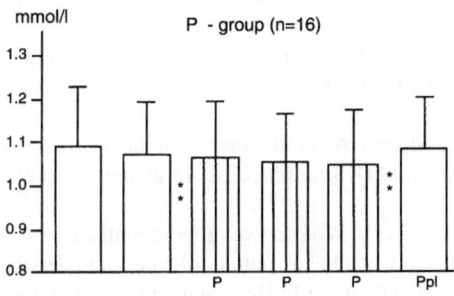

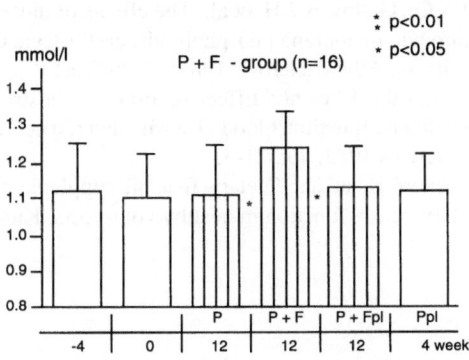

Fig. 5. HDL-cholesterol in patients with mild essential hypertension randomized to fish oil (group F), propranolol (group P) and to propranolol in combination with fish oil (group P + F), pl = placebo.

pattern that further reduces coronary risk. Thus treatment with n-3 fatty acids is recommended in patients with mild hypertension.

References

1. Singer P., Wirth M., Voigt S. et al.: Blood pressure- and lipid-lowering effect of mackerel and herring diet in patients with mild essential hypertension. Atherosclerosis 1985; 56:223-235

2. Knapp H.R., FitzGerald G.A.: The antihypertensive effects of fish oil: a controlled study of polyunsaturated fatty acid supplements in essential hypertension. New. Engl. J. Med. 1989; 320:1037-1043

3. v. Schacky C., Fischer S., Weber P.C.: Long-term effects of dietary marine omega-3 fatty acids upon plasma and cellular lipids, platelet function, and eicosanoid formation in humans. J. Clin. Invest. 1985; 76:1626-1631

4. Singer P., Jaeger W., Wirth M. et al.: Lipid and blood pressure-lowering effect of mackerel diet in man. Atherosclerosis 1983; 49:99-108

5. Urakaze M., Hanasaki N., Hamazaki T. et al.: Effects of fish oil concentrate on blood pressure of mild essential hypertensives (abstract). 8th International Symposium on Atherosclerosis, Rome, 1988, p 974

6. Lorenz R., Sprengler U., Fischer S. et al.: Platelet function, thromboxane formation and blood pressure control during supplementation of the Western diet with cod liver oil. Circulation 1983; 67:504-511

7. Knapp H.R., Gregory D., Nolan S.: Dietary polyunsaturates, vascular function and prostaglandins: In Galli C, Simopoulos AP (Eds): *Dietary n-3 and n-6 Fatty Acids*, New York, Plenun, 1989, pp 283-295.

8. Locker R., Sachinidis A., Steiner A. et al.: Fischol antagonisiert den Angiotensin II(AII) - induzierten Phosphatidylinositol (IP) Stoffwechsel in glatten Muskelzellen. Hochdruck 1988; 8:49

9. Haller H., Passfall J., Bock A. et al.: Wirkung von Eicosapentaensaure (EPA) auf Blutdruck und intrazellulares freies Calcium (Ca^{++}) bei essentieller Hypertonie. Hochdruck 1987; 8:V2

10. Jørgensen A.K., Nielsen A.H., Dyerberg J.: Hemostatic factors and renin in Greenland Eskimos on a high eicosapentaenoic acid intake. Acta Med. Scand. 1986; 219:473-479

11. Cartwright I.J., Pockley A.G., Galloway J.H. et al.: The effects of dietary omega-3 polyunsaturated fatty acids on erythrocyte membrane phospholipids, erythrocyte deformability and blood viscosity in healthy volunteers. Atherosclerosis 1985; 55:267-281

12. Terano T., Hirai A., Hamazaki T. et al.: Effect of oral administration of highly purified eicosapentaenoic acid on platelet function, blood viscosity and red cell deformability in healthy human subjects. Atherosclerosis 1983; 46:321-331

13. Dusing R., Struck A., Scherf H. et al.: Dietary fish oil supplementation: Effects on renal hemodynamics and renal excretory function in healthy volunteers. Kidney Int. 1987; 31:268

Subject Index

I

L

M